Workbook to Accompany
Thomson Delmar Learning's
ADMINISTRATIVE
MEDICAL ASSISTING
Third Edition

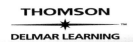

THOMSON
DELMAR LEARNING

Workbook to Accompany

Thomson Delmar Learning's

ADMINISTRATIVE MEDICAL ASSISTING

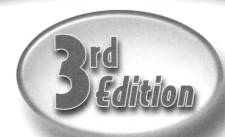

3rd Edition

Prepared by

Barbara M. Dahl,

CMA, CPC

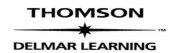

THOMSON

DELMAR LEARNING

**Workbook to Accompany Thomson Delmar Learning's
Administrative Medical Assisting, Third Edition**
Prepared by Barbara M. Dahl

**Vice President, Health Care
Business Unit:**
William Brottmiller

Editorial Director:
Matthew Kane

Acquisitions Editor:
Rhonda Dearborn

Developmental Editor:
Sarah Duncan

Editorial Assistant:
Debra Gorgos

Marketing Director:
Jennifer McAvey

Marketing Coordinator:
Kimberly Duffy

Technology Director:
Laurie K. Davis

Technology Project Manager:
Mary Colleen Liburdi

Technology Project Coordinator:
Carolyn Fox

Production Director:
Carolyn Miller

Production Manager:
Barbara A. Bullock

Production Editor:
Jack Pendleton

Project Editor:
Natalle Pashoukos

NOTICE TO THE READER

Publisher does not warrant or guarantee any of the products described herein or perform any independent analysis in connection with any of the product information contained herein. Publisher does not assume, and expressly disclaims, any obligation to obtain and include information other than that provided to it by the manufacturer.

The reader is expressly warned to consider and adopt all safety precautions that might be indicated by the activities described herein and to avoid all potential hazards. By following the instructions contained herein, the reader willingly assumes all risks in connection with such instructions.

The publisher makes no representations or warranties of any kind, including but not limited to, the warranties of fitness for particular purpose or merchantability, nor are any such representations implied with respect to the material set forth herein, and the publisher takes no responsibility with respect to such material. The publisher shall not be liable for any special, consequential, or exemplary damages resulting, in whole or part, from the reader's use of, or reliance upon, this material.

Contents

To the Learner

This workbook is part of a dynamic learning system that will help reinforce the essential competencies you need to enter the field of medical assisting and become a successful, multiskilled medical assistant. It has been completely revised to challenge you to apply the chapter knowledge from *Thomson Delmar Learning's Administrative Medical Assisting, Third Edition,* to develop basic competencies, use critical thinking skills, and integrate your knowledge effectively.

WORKBOOK ORGANIZATION

The workbook chapters are divided into the following sections: Chapter Pre-Test, Performance Objectives, Vocabulary Builder, Learning Review, Certification Review, Case Study, Self-Assessment, and Chapter Post-Test. Each chapter also contains checklists for evaluation of chapter knowledge, certification criteria, and competency assessments.

The content of the workbook has been conceived to give you a creative and interpretive forum to apply the knowledge you have learned, not simply to repeat information to answer questions. Realistic simulations appear throughout the workbook referencing characters referred to in the textbook. This gives the material a real-world feel that comes as close as possible to your future experiences in an ambulatory setting.

CHECKLISTS

Evaluation of Chapter Knowledge sheets are incorporated at the end of each chapter to review theoretical understanding and define competency while at the same time incorporating essential interpersonal communication and professional skills. The assessment and grading of these sheets is done by self-evaluation.

Certification Criteria Checklists are provided at the end of each chapter to help you track your progress in learning the content covered on the certification examinations from AAMA and AMT. As you complete each chapter of the text and workbook, use the Certification Criteria Checklists and checklists at the end of the workbook to highlight the examination criteria covered in that chapter. The checklists correlate to each of the three examinations: CMA, RMA, CMAS.

Competency Assessment Checklists are designed to set criteria or standards that should be observed while a specific procedure is being performed. They follow the same procedural steps as listed in the textbook. As you perform each procedure, the evaluation section of this checklist can be used to judge your performance. The instructor will use this checklist to evaluate your competency in performing this skill. A master Competency Assessment Tracking Sheet is also provided for you in the front of the workbook to use as an overview of all competency assessment checklists in the workbook. This tracking sheet can serve as a table of contents for all checklists, as well as a guide to easily view your performance on the assessment checklists.

The format of the Competency Assessment Checklists is designed to provide specific conditions, standards, skill steps, and evaluation and documentation sections for essential skills necessary for an entry-level medical assistant.

MEDICAL OFFICE SIMULATION SOFTWARE

Six case studies are found in Appendix A of this workbook. They are designed to give you experience using practice management software in performing some of the tasks that medical assistants complete on a daily basis.

Medical Office Simulation Software (MOSS) is a highly interactive medical practice management software CD-ROM included with the workbook. MOSS includes eight basic components, common to most practice management software, including Patient Registration, Appointment Scheduling, Procedure Posting, Insurance Billing, Posting Payments, Patient Billing, Report Generation, and File Maintenance.

Refer to Appendix A in the workbook for setup and usage instructions to install MOSS on your computer.

FINAL THOUGHTS

- Feel certain that each procedure and concept you master is an important step toward preparing your skills and knowledge for the workplace. The textbook, student software CD, and workbook have all been coordinated to meet the core objectives. Review the performance objectives at the beginning of each chapter in the workbook before you begin to study; they are a road map that will take you to your goals.

- Remember that you are the learner, so you can take credit for your success. The instructor is an important guide on this journey, and the text, workbook, student software CD, and externships are tools, but whether or not you use the tools wisely is ultimately up to you.

- Evaluate yourself and your study habits. Take positive steps toward improving yourself, and avoid habits that could limit your success. For example, do you let family responsibilities or social opportunities interfere with your study? If so, sit down with your family and plan a schedule for study that they will support and to which you will adhere. Find a special place to study that is free from distraction.

- Because regulations vary from state to state regarding which procedures can be performed by a medical assistant, it will be important to check specific regulations in your state. A medical assistant should never perform any procedure without being aware of legal responsibilities, correct procedure, and proper authorization.

Enjoy your career in medical assisting!

Competency Assessment Tracking Sheet

Student Name: _____

Procedure Number and Title	Date Assessment Completed and Competency Achieved			
	School Date/Initials	Externship Date/Initials	Externship Date/Initials	Externship Date/Initials
EXAMPLE:				
13-1 Checking In Patients	2/23/XX MP	3/15/XX BG	4/20/XX SD	5/1/XX JP
9-1 Control of Bleeding				
9-2 Applying an Arm Splint				
9-3 Abdominal Thrusts for a Conscious Adult				
9-4 Abdominal Thrusts for an Unconscious Adult or Child				
9-5 Abdominal Thrusts for a Conscious Child				
9-6 Back Blows and Chest Thrusts for a Conscious Infant Who Is Choking				
9-7 Back Blows and Chest Thrusts for an Unconscious Infant				
9-8 Rescue Breathing for Adults				
9-9 Rescue Breathing for Children				
9-10 Rescue Breathing for Infants				
9-11 CPR for Adults				
9-12 CPR for Children				
9-13 CPR for Infants				
11-1 Software Installation				
11-2 Hardware Installation				
12-1 Answering and Screening Incoming Calls				
12-2 Transferring a Call				
12-3 Taking a Telephone Message				
12-4 Handling Problem Calls				
12-5 Placing Outgoing Calls				
12-6 Recording a Telephone Message on an Answering Device or Voice Mail System				
13-1 Checking In Patients and Sharing Office Policies				
13-2 Cancellation Procedures				
13-3 Establishing the Appointment Matrix				
13-4 Scheduling of Inpatient and Outpatient Admissions and Procedures				
13-5 Making an Appointment on the Telephone				
14-1 Steps for Manual Filing with a Numeric System				
14-2 Steps for Manual Filing with a Subject Filing System				
14-3 Correcting a Paper Medical Record				
14-4 Correcting an Electronic Medical Record				
14-5 Establishing a Paper Medical Chart for a New Patient				

Procedure Number and Title	Date Assessment Completed and Competency Achieved			
	School Date/Initials	Externship Date/Initials	Externship Date/Initials	Externship Date/Initials
15-1 Preparing and Composing Business Correspondence Using All Components (Computerized Approach)				
15-2 Addressing Envelopes According to United States Postal Regulations				
15-3 Folding Letters for Standard Envelopes				
15-4 Creating a Mass Mailing Using Mail Merge				
15-5 Preparing Outgoing Mail According to United States Postal Regulations				
15-6 Preparing, Sending, and Receiving a Fax				
17-1 Recording/Posting Patient Charges, Payments, and Adjustments				
17-2 Balancing Day Sheets in a Manual System				
17-3 Preparing a Deposit				
17-4 Reconciling a Bank Statement				
17-5 Balancing Petty Cash				
17-6 Recording a Nonsufficient Funds Check				
18-1 Screening for Insurance				
18-2 Obtaining Referrals and Authorizations				
19-1 Current Procedural Terminology Coding				
19-2 International Classification of Diseases, 9th Revision, Clinical Modificaiton Coding				
19-3 Applying Third-Party Guidelines				
19-4 Completing a Medicare CMS-1500 Claim Form				
20-1 Explaining Fees in the First Telephone Interview				
20-2 Prepare Itemized Patient Accounts for Billing				
20-3 Post/Record Adjustments and refunds including Collection Agency Payments				
21-1 Preparing Accounts Receivable Trial Balance				
22-1 Preparing a Meeting Agenda				
22-2 Supervising a Student Practicum				
22-3 Making Travel Arrangements				
22-4 Making Travel Arrangements via the Internet				
22-5 Developing and Maintaining a Procedure Manual				
23-1 Develop and Maintain a Policy Manual				
23-2 Prepare a Job Description				
23-3 Conduct Interviews				
23-4 Orient Personnel				

Workbook to Accompany

Thomson Delmar Learning's

ADMINISTRATIVE

MEDICAL ASSISTING

Third Edition

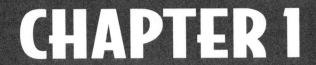

CHAPTER 1

Medical Assisting as a Profession

CHAPTER PRE-TEST

Perform this test without looking at the book. This is just to see how well you have understood and can recall the information in this chapter after you have read it, but before you have completed the workbook exercises. You will not be graded on this portion (other than the grade you give yourself). Justify any "false" answers.

1. Are medical assistants licensed, registered, or certified? (circle all that apply)

2. Anyone can take the national (AAMA) medical assisting examination without going to a special program. (T or F)

3. Medical assistants are only allowed to work in the back office. (T or F)

4. Medical assistants can become office managers. (T or F)

5. Medical assistants work as medical receptionists, medical bookkeepers, medical insurance coders and billers, transcriptionists, office managers, laboratory assistants, surgery assistants, and clinical assistants. (circle all that apply)

6. Choosing to attend an accredited medical assisting program is not as important as getting trained as quickly as possible so you can get a job. (T or F)

7. Medical assistants do not have to be credentialed to work in the field. (T or F)

INTRODUCTION

Medical assisting is a fairly conservative career that requires many professional traits. Professionalism includes things such as mature work ethics, attitude, and behaviors.

Your appearance is also an important part of professionalism. When you come to work, make sure you are dressed appropriately in clean, pressed scrubs (do not forget about clean shoes!), with clean, well-kept hair, and clean, clipped, unpolished nails. Use good personal hygiene and keep your teeth in good health. Your clothes and personal appearance should look clean, fresh, and healthy. Your appearance sets the tone for the office. If you want to wear jewelry and makeup, make sure the jewelry is small and do not wear rings other than your engagement and wedding rings. Makeup should be conservative and natural looking. Wear deodorant, but not perfume.

Your work ethics should include coming to work on time and showing responsibility for performing your job well. Sometimes we forget that we are being paid for every minute of our time spent at work and our physician–employers deserve value for their money. We should stay busy at work and work hard for our employers. Your professional ethics include using proper language, treating all your patients and coworkers with respect, and being helpful and cheerful.

Other parts of professionalism include obtaining and maintaining your credentials and certificates, continuing your education, being actively involved in your professional organizations, and networking with other medical assistants. Chapter 24 of your textbook more completely covers these attributes.

Personal attributes of a medical assistant include traits such as empathy, dependability, initiative, flexibility, desire to learn, ability to communicate (written and orally), and, of course, professionalism. These attributes are covered individually in your textbook.

How we treat people—our patients, coworkers, employers, other members of the health care team, and the general public—helps us form our professional behaviors and demeanor. We need to learn to treat all people with respect, empathy, impartial behavior, tact, and diplomacy, without judgment. Remember, as a medical assistant, you are a professional.

PERFORMANCE OBJECTIVES

After successful completion of this chapter, you should be able to list and justify professional attributes and personal traits required of medical assistants. You should be able to explain the difference between accreditation, certification, receiving a certificate or diploma, and licensure, and to compare the Certified Medical Assistant (CMA) with the Registered Medical Assistant (RMA) credentials as far as educational and training requirements. You also should be familiar with the two main medical assisting program accrediting organizations, Accrediting Bureau of Health Education Schools (ABHES) and Commission on Accreditation of Allied Health Education Programs (CAAHEP). In addition, you should know how to treat people and how to act and look like a professional. Try not to look back at the introductory section of this workbook as you complete the following exercise. If necessary, reread the Introduction. *The following statements are related to your learning objectives for this chapter. Fill in the blanks with the appropriate term(s):*

To be a good medical assistant you will need to acquire many (1) _____ traits. These traits include mature (2) _____ _____, (3) _____ and (4) _____. (5) _____ also is important. Your scrubs should be (6) _____ and (7) _____. Your personal appearance should be (8) _____, (9) _____, and (10) _____. If you wear jewelry or makeup, the jewelry should be (11) _____ and the makeup should be (12) _____ and (13) _____ _____. Wear (14) _____ but not (15) _____. Work ethics should include (16) _____ and showing (17) _____ _____ your job well. Our physician–employers deserve (18) _____ for their money, and we provide that by (19) _____ and (20) _____. Professional ethical behaviors include (21) _____, (22) _____, and being (23) _____ and (24) _____. As a professional medical assistant, you should obtain and maintain your (25) _____ and (26) _____ and continue your

(27) _____. You should become actively involved in your (28) _____

_____ and (29) _____ with other medical assistants.

You should strive to obtain personal attributes such as (30) _____,

(31) _____, (32) _____, (33) _____,

(34) _____, (35) _____, and of course,

(36) _____. Treat all people with (37) _____, (38) _____,

(39) _____, (40) _____, and (41) _____.

VOCABULARY BUILDER

Find the words below that are misspelled; circle them, and then correctly spell them in the spaces provided. Then replace the highlighted words in the following paragraph with the correct vocabulary terms from the list. (Be sure to spell them all correctly!)

acredits	complience	integrate
ambulatory care setting	credential	liscensed
attributes	disposition	licensure
associate's	empathy	litiguous
certify	facilitates	practicums
competancy	improvising	versatile

_____   _____   _____

_____   _____

The medical assistant is a **multiskilled** (1) _____ health care professional

who performs many clinical and administrative duties in physicians' offices and **outpatient facilities**

(2) _____. In today's **lawsuit-prone** (3) _____

society, health care consumers are demanding educated, skilled health care professionals. The

American Association of Medical Assistants is a national organization that **recognizes qualifying**

standards for (4) _____ medical assisting education programs and

practical applications of theory (5) _____; provides national **proficiency**

(6) _____ examinations that **guarantee** (7) _____

the skills of medical assistants at entry-level job, earning them the **official credit** (8) _____

_____ of CMA; and encourages continuing education. Medical assistants are

educated at community, junior, and technical colleges and proprietary schools in programs that

are in **agreement** (9) _____ with essential guidelines and stan-

dards, and they sometimes earn **2-year** (10) _____ college degrees.

The medical assistant must **combine** (11) _____ several **characteristics**

(12) _____ that will enhance a professional appearance and attitude. Several

of these include a warm and friendly **temperament** (13) _____ that **allows**

for easy (14) _____ communication, **an insight into another's feelings or**

emotions (15) _____, and a talent for **performing without previous**

preparation (16) _____ good solutions to unexpected situations. Medical assistants work with **legally authorized to practice** (17) _____ medical and nursing professionals, who have gone through a process of **granting of licenses to practice** (18) _____.

From the vocabulary list below, select the term that best fits the sentences.

accreditation   certification examination   competency
CMA   credentialed   diploma
license   RMA

Medical Assisting Programs undergo (1) _____ processes that prove they are covering the right curriculum and properly serving the education/training needs of their students. Included in this process is proof that each required (2) _____ has been assessed.

When you graduate from your medical assisting program, you will be given a (3) _____ (sometimes called a certificate), which proves that you have taken all the courses necessary to graduate from the program.

After taking and passing a national (4) _____ examination offered by either AAMA or AMT, you will be (5) _____ as either an (6) _____ or a (7) _____.

None of the above documents or processes should be confused with having a (8) _____, which requires a state-mandated scope of practice.

Word Game

Find the words in the grid below. They may go in any direction. The first four lines of unused letters contain a hidden message.

```
B L E C O M E C E R T I F I E D Z B E C G O
M I P I H S N R E T X E E I N L I C E N S E
V T O L V E D Q Y C N E T E P M O C I C O S
N I T C I N I U E E L E A R N I N T G S Z I
B G C L E E T N Z M Z W Q M Z K T K H C P V
M I D H J R C L T R P Y V M T E K D L O R O
N O L T X X T N G E R A F Q S A R M R P O R
O U D V N K L I A G G A T E B R M D N E F P
I S W Z G N C L F I C R R H J R E O Q O E M
T P J R W M F X J I L A A G Y L R D L F S I
A R J K A M K B L P C P X T A F W D D P S L
T R L Y X R J I I Y P A M I E B P I E R I N
I D B R R X T H R R M Z T O K R T S T A O D
D T J V R A S O A Y T N P I C Q M P A C N Y
E R T Q T N T C K P E W N C O C C O V T A V
R F K E R A T T P D Z K P R W N Z S I I L Y
C Z W E L I R V E F N D G F K L M I T C I F
C Y T U C M W R X K Q P N A D N Z T L E S N
A N B U L T C T N H L K N R M R T I U D M V
I M M T T R W R N D H K V M R R Z O C J M R
A M B Y H A T T R I B U T E V Y D N Z Q K Z
G D E X T E R I T Y Y R A T E I R P O R P K
```

accreditation
ambulatory care setting
attribute
certified
CMA
competency
compliance
credentialed
cultivate

dexterity
diploma
disposition
empathy
externship
facilitate
improvise
integrate
internship

license
litigious
practicum
professionalism
proprietary
RMA
scope of practice

LEARNING REVIEW

True or False

Mark true statements with a T and false statements with an F. Then rewrite each false statement to make it true.

_____ 1. Medical assistants are licensed by each state. _____

_____ 2. All medical assisting programs are accredited by either CAAHEP or ABHES. _____
_____

_____ 3. Anyone can call themselves a medical assistant, but professional medical assistants have graduated from an accredited program and obtained a credential to prove their competency. _____

_____ 4. If you graduate from a medical assisting program and get a diploma or certificate, then you are automatically credentialed. _____

_____ 5. Medical assistants continue their education by attending seminars, workshops, and professional meetings. _____

_____ 6. Both RMAs and CMAs are required to obtain continuing education units (CEUs) to recertify. _____

_____ 7. Medical assistants must be either a CMA or an RMA to join the AAMA or the AMT.
_____

_____ 8. The AAMA "owns" the CMA credential, and no person may call themselves a CMA unless they have passed the national AAMA Certification Examination. _____
_____

Matching

A. externship
B. scope of practice
C. mandatory
D. voluntary
E. continuing education units

1. Recertification as a CMA may be obtained by either retaking the examination or obtaining _____.

2. Going into a medical setting to practice skills while still a student is called _____.

3. A description of a health care professional's job and legal boundaries is called a _____.

4. Certification and registration as a CMA/RMA is still _____.

5. Licensure is _____ for many professions.

Fill in the Blanks

Medical assistants learn a variety of clinical, administrative, and general skills in their courses. Write a C next to each clinical course, an A next to each administrative course, and a G next to each general course.

1. Medical Records _____

2. Therapeutic Relations _____

3. Medical Law & Ethics _____

4. Medical Computers _____

5. Pathology _____

6. Transcription _____

7. Coding and Insurance _____

8. Receptioning _____

9. Ambulatory Surgery _____

10. Anatomy and Physiology _____

11. Pharmacology _____

12. Laboratory Procedures _____

13. Terminology _____

14. Taking Vital Signs _____

15. Write the name, address, phone number, and Web site address for the AAMA. _____

_____

16. Write the name, address, phone number, and Web site address for the AMT. _____

_____

17. Name the nine personal attributes of a professional medical assistant. Then, for each attribute, write a sentence that describes how possessing it contributes to better patient care and good relationships with coworkers and employers.

(1) _____

_____

_____

(2) _____

_____

_____

(3) _____

_____

_____

(4) _____

_____

_____

(5) _____

_____

_____

(6) _____

_____

_____

(7) _____

_____

_____

(8) _____

_____

_____

(9) _____

_____

_____

18. Name four reasons why the medical assisting profession has grown to require more formal, skilled education and credentialing for medical assistants.

(1) _____

_____

(2) _____

_____

(3) _____

_____

(4) _____

_____

19. The U. S. Department of Labor, Bureau of Statistics, lists medical assisting as the fastest growing allied health profession. Name eight settings where medical assistants are usually employed.

(1) _____ (5) _____

(2) _____ (6) _____

(3) _____ (7) _____

(4) _____ (8) _____

Choose the Correct Answer

1. *Circle the two correct responses.* Medical assistants must recertify their credential every five years. The two ways to recertify for the CMA credential are:

   a. Accumulate approved continuing education hours.

   b. Obtain a good recommendation from a physician–employer.

   c. Become licensed.

   d. Retake the certification examination.

2. *Circle the two correct responses.* The Role Delineation Components is a list of competencies compiled by practicing medical assistants. These competencies are used by medical assisting program directors to develop curricula that ensure:

   a. certification

   b. employment preparedness

   c. continuing education

   d. high-quality medical assisting education

3. A system of values that each individual has that determines perceptions of right and wrong is called:

   a. laws

   b. ethics

   c. attributes

   d. attitudes

4. Stepping into a patient's place, discovering what the patient is experiencing, then recognizing and identifying with those feelings is:

   a. sympathy

   b. association

   c. flexibility

   d. empathy

5. Recertification of the CMA credential must be undertaken every:

   a. year

   b. six months

   c. seven years

   d. five years

6. Courses in a professional medical assisting program include a complement of general knowledge classes such as anatomy and physiology and:

   a. assisting with minor surgery

   b. CPR

   c. medical terminology

   d. computer applications

7. The type of regulation for health care providers that is legislated by each state and is mandatory to practice is:

   a. licensure

   b. registration

   c. certification

   d. a and c

CERTIFICATION REVIEW

The following questions are designed to mimic the certification examinations. You can use these questions like a small "Certification Examination Study Guide," but this is not meant to take the place of the more extensive study guides. Use this section to determine where to concentrate your efforts when studying for the certification examination.

1. Medical assistants may take the AAMA examination to obtain which credential?
   a. CMAS
   b. RMA
   c. CMA
   d. CPC
   e. AMT

2. Select the following statement that best describes the professional medical assistant.
   a. has good written and oral communication skills
   b. looks and acts professional at all times
   c. is aware of her or his scope of practice and stays within her or his legal boundaries
   d. assists the physician in all areas of the ambulatory care setting
   e. all of the above

3. Good medical assistants portray their professional attitude by:
   a. discussing their personal lives at work because it is therapeutic for them
   b. gossiping with their coworkers to help them with their problems
   c. reminding their physicians that they only work 7.5 hours per day
   d. helping patients in a friendly and empathetic manner
   e. being too busy to do more than the basic workload

4. To become involved with their professional organization, medical assistants could:
   a. attend local chapter or state meetings
   b. attend a national conference or state convention
   c. join their national organization
   d. offer to serve on a local, state, or national committee
   e. all of the above

CASE STUDIES

Case 1

During your course of studies to become a medical assistant, you volunteer to help out at a multi-doctor urgent care center in the center of a large city to gain some firsthand experience in a professional setting.

Discuss the following issues:
1. What about this opportunity is interesting to you to the extent that you want to volunteer in a professional setting?
2. Even though you are a volunteer, why is it important to look and behave like a professional? What does this entail?
3. You ask the CMA if you can be allowed to watch the performance of some basic clinical procedures. The CMA must get permission from the center's office manager and physician and obtain the consent of the patient. Why are these permissions necessary? How are patients' rights affected by your request?
4. After volunteering at the urgent care center for a period of time, you decide to try volunteering in another setting to get a new experience. How are your personal interests and goals important in choosing the right setting? Why are different personal qualities and ambitions needed in each setting; for example, how does a hospital setting differ from a medical laboratory?

Case 2

You are scheduled to go for your yearly complete physical examination. You decide to use this as an opportunity to study an ambulatory care setting.

Consider the following:
1. How is a patient's first impression of the physician's office and staff important in establishing a good relationship between the patient and the health care professionals who work there?
2. What, if anything, would you change about the experience to make it more successful from the patient's point of view?
3. Describe how the CMA at the physician's office interacted with patients. How did the CMA interact with the other health care professionals there? What kind of duties did the CMA perform?

Case 3

Michelle Lucas is preparing for externship. Michelle is an excellent student, detail oriented, responsible, and professional in her dress and attitude. Michelle is eager to do her externship with a large general practice or clinic with open hours built into the schedule for emergency patients, such as Inner City Health Care. Michelle is intrigued by the idea of working with a group of physicians and a diverse patient population where she can really work on improving her triage skills. Michelle, however, is shy and quiet; she has difficulty meeting new people and relies on a core group of friends.

Discuss the following:
1. Is Michelle really suited to externship at Inner City Health Care? What are the potential advantages or disadvantages of this externship placement?
2. Consider your own short- and long-range goals. How important is it to challenge yourself, personally and professionally, with experiences that contribute to your growth and knowledge? How can you use your externship placement to work toward fulfilling your goals?

SELF-ASSESSMENT

1. As you begin your education as a medical assistant, you may not be sure whether you want to work in the administrative and clerical area or in the clinical and laboratory areas. What are some ways for you to explore the various options?

2. For each of the personal attributes used in your textbook to describe a professional, identify individuals from your family, friends, work, or community who possess one or more of those traits. Explain why you chose them.

3. Imagine your first day in your externship. What will you wear? How will you prepare the night before? Would you change anything about your hairstyle? Makeup? Jewelry?

CHAPTER POST-TEST

This test is similar to the Pre-Test. Perform this test without looking at the book. This is just to see how well you have understood and can recall the information presented in this chapter after you have studied it and completed the workbook exercises. You will not be graded on this portion (other than the grade you give yourself), but this is an excellent preparation for your instructor's test. You may use this Post-Test to determine what areas you need to study more. Justify any "false" answers.

1. Medical assistants may be either licensed, registered, or certified. (T or F)

2. The AAMA medical assisting certification examination is available to anyone, even people who have not been formally trained. (T or F)

3. Medical assistants only work in the clerical parts of the office. (T or F)

4. The position of Office Manager is a career option for a medical assistant. (T or F)

5. Medical assistants work as medical receptionists, medical bookkeepers, medical insurance coders and billers, transcriptionists, office managers, laboratory assistants, surgery assistants, and clinical assistants. (circle all that apply)

6. Getting trained as quickly as possible is more important than attending an accredited medical assisting program. (T or F)

7. Medical assistants may work in their field even without being credentialed. (T or F)

EVALUATION OF CHAPTER KNOWLEDGE

Evaluate your achievements.

Skills	Student Self-Evaluation		
	Good	Average	Poor
Attendance/punctuality	____	____	____
Personal appearance	____	____	____
Effort applied	____	____	____
Self-motivation	____	____	____
Courteous behavior	____	____	____
Positive attitude	____	____	____
Assignments completed on time	____	____	____
Professionalism	____	____	____

Skills	Student Self-Evaluation		
	Good	Average	Poor
I understand externship opportunities available to me.	____	____	____
I understand requirements of the externship as a component of the requirements needed for graduation from an accredited education program.	____	____	____
I recognize and apply concepts of performance objectives in setting and achieving my goals.	____	____	____

CHAPTER 2

Health Care Settings and the Health Care Team

CHAPTER PRE-TEST

Perform this test without looking at the book. This is just to see how well you have understood and can recall the information in this chapter after you have read it, but before you have completed the workbook exercises. You will not be graded on this portion (other than the grade you give yourself). Justify any "false" answers.

1. Doctors who work in sole proprietorships work alone and employ no other doctors. (T or F)

2. Two doctors make up a partnership, and three doctors make up a corporation. (T or F)

3. Urgent care centers are like emergency rooms and do not offer routine well-patient services. (T or F)

4. Medical assistants do not generally work in urgent care centers. (T or F)

5. Managed care may set limits on the services your doctor can provide to a patient. (T or F)

6. Physicians are licensed to practice nationally so they can move freely from state to state. (T or F)

7. Doctors of chiropractic medicine work only on the musculoskeletal systems. (T or F)

8. Acupuncturists treat pain and a variety of disorders in the gastrointestinal urogenital, gynecologic, circulatory, respiratory, neuromusculoskeletal, and many other systems. (T or F)

INTRODUCTION

The medical assistant is one member of a dynamic, growing health care industry. As medical settings evolve to meet the challenges of technology and societal needs, the medical assistant represents a vital link in the health care team and is responsible for many duties, both clinical and administrative. Students beginning a course of study to become a medical assistant can use this workbook chapter to understand the medical settings where medical assistants are employed, learn about the shift of the health care industry toward managed care, and discover the wide range of health care professionals the medical assistant comes into contact with in various medical settings.

PERFORMANCE OBJECTIVES

After successful completion of this chapter, you should be able to list four or more physician specialists, at least three alternative health care specialists, and five allied health professionals. You should understand the differences in education and training between medical assistants and nurses and the different levels of nursing. You also should be able to define health maintenance organizations (HMOs), preferred provider organizations (PPOs), independent physician associations (IPAs), and managed care plans, including their purposes, limitations, and benefits. Try not to look back at the textbook as you fill in the blanks in the following paragraphs. *The following statements are related to your learning objectives for this chapter. Fill in the blanks with the appropriate term(s):*

Originally, (1) _____ were designed to serve patients more efficiently and effectively while cutting costs. Critics charge that patients under HMO plans are often denied many services because they are not considered (2) _____. Physicians have joined together to form large (3) _____ to control costs within their practices. Controlling costs also has caused many insurers to direct dollars away from hospitals and toward (4) _____ care.

The medical assistant works directly under the supervision of the physician and serves as an important link between the physician and the (5) _____. Although nurses are educated and trained to work in (6) _____, extended care facilities, and inpatient settings, many do work side by side with medical assistants in the clinic setting.

Alternative therapies, which include biofeedback, hypnotherapy, aromatherapy, massage therapy, and (7) _____, are widely accepted.

VOCABULARY BUILDER

Find the words below that are misspelled; circle them, and then correctly spell them in the spaces provided. Then insert the correct vocabulary terms from the list that best fit the descriptions below.

A. accupuncture
C. health maintainance organizations (HMOs)
E. independent physician association (IPA)
G. prefered provider organization (PPO)
I. triage

B. frindge benefits
D. intagrative medicine
F. managed care operations
H. ambulatory care settings
J. homeopathy

_____   _____   _____

_____   _____

1.____ Organizations designed to provide a full range of health care services under one roof, or, more recently, through a network of participating physicians within a defined geographic area

2.____ Advantages added to the terms of employment, such as health insurance and vacation time

3.____ An independent organization of physicians, whose members agree to treat patients for an agreed-on fee

4.____ The theory that large doses of drugs that produce symptoms of a disease in healthy people will cure the symptoms when given in small amounts

5.____ This kind of medical setting includes environments such as a medical office, an urgent or primary care center, and a managed care organization

6.____ A nontraditional medical approach proving to be effective in treating drug dependency and managing pain that requires insertion of needles at specified sites of the body

7.____ Organizations in which physicians network to offer discounts to employers and other purchasers of health care

8.____ Alternative forms of health care increasingly perceived as complements to traditional health care

9.____ Determine priorities for medical action and assess patient needs

10.____ A standard of patient care that seeks to provide quality care while containing costs

LEARNING REVIEW

1. How has managed care changed medical settings as the health care profession works to offer high-quality, cost-effective care to patients? What is the medical assistant's role in contributing to the efforts of the health care team in an era of managed care?

_____

_____

_____

_____

_____

_____

2. For each of the three forms of medical practice management, list appropriate medical settings. Then describe the patient's experience with care under each form of medical practice management. Note how patient experiences may differ and why this is possible.

Sole Proprietorships:

A. Medical settings _____

_____

B. Patient experience _____

_____

_____

Partnerships:

A. Medical settings _____

_____

B. Patient experience _____

_____

_____

Corporations:

A. Medical settings _____

_____

B. Patient experience _____

_____

_____

3. Name three ways in which insurers, providers, and patients are working creatively to meet the challenge of managed care to keep costs down.

(1) _____

_____

_____

(2) _____

_____

_____

(3) _____

_____

_____

4. A. Name six administrative duties of the medical assistant as a member of the health care team.

(1) _____ (4) _____

(2) _____ (5) _____

(3) _____ (6) _____

B. Name five clinical duties of the medical assistant as a member of the health care team.

(1) _____

(2) _____

(3) _____

(4) _____

(5) _____

5. A. In the medical field, the abbreviation *Dr.* is used and the title *doctor* is addressed to the person qualified by education, training, and licensure to practice medicine. List the medical degree associated with each of the following credentials, and define each specialty.

MD _____

_____

_____

DPM _____

_____

_____

DC _____

_____

_____

ND _____

_____

_____

DO _____

_____

_____

OD _____

_____

_____

DDS _____

_____

_____

B. Using a medical dictionary or encyclopedia to help you, define the following six medical and surgical specialists. Refer to your textbook for a complete listing of medical and surgical specialties.

(1) Radiation oncologist _____

_____

_____

(2) Obstetrician/gynecologist _____

_____

_____

(3) Neurologist _____

_____

_____

(4) Gerontologist _____

_____

_____

(5) Ophthalmologist _____

_____

_____

(6) Pediatrician _____

_____

_____

6. Medical assistants are only one of many allied health and other health care professionals who form the health care team. Although medical assistants may not work directly with each professional, they are likely to come into contact with many of them through telephone, written, or electronic communication. List six of those types of professionals.

(1) _____

(2) _____

(3) _____

(4) _____

(5) _____

(6) _____

7. In an effort to receive alternative therapies, many health care providers and patients are pursuing integrative medicine as a complement to traditional health care. Name seven alternative forms of health care that may be currently perceived to supplement traditional health care.

(1) _____

(2) _____

(3) _____

(4) _____

(5) _____

(6) _____

(7) _____

CERTIFICATION REVIEW

These questions are designed to mimic the certification examinations. You can use these questions like a small "Certification Examination Study Guide," but this is not meant to take the place of the more extensive study guides. Use this portion to determine where to concentrate your efforts when studying for the certification examination.

1. The form of medical practice management that states that personal property cannot be attached in litigation is a:

a. partnership

b. sole proprietorship

c. corporation

d. group practice

2. The minimum amount of time it takes to become an MD without specialization is:

    a. 6 years

    b. 9 years

    c. 12 years

    d. 4 years

3. Critical care medicine and pain management may require subspecialty certificates to practice:

    a. anesthesiology

    b. family practice

    c. pathology

    d. radiology

4. The American Society of Clinical Pathology is the professional organization that oversees credentialing and education in what allied health area?

    a. nurses

    b. medical laboratory

    c. registered dietitian

    d. physical therapy

5. The specialty that treats patients using the relationship between mind, body, spirit, and nature is called:

    a. chiropractic

    b. osteopathy

    c. podiatry

    d. naturopathy

CASE STUDIES

In each of the following scenarios, consider the following: (1) How can the patients be encouraged to consider themselves as a part of the health care team? and (2) What is the role of the medical assistant?

Abigail Johnson is an older woman in her 70s with mature-onset diabetes. She is having trouble managing her diet; she lives alone but craves social contact and seems to enjoy her visits to the family physician's office.

Herb Fowler is an African-American man in his early 50s. Herb is a heavy smoker, is significantly overweight, and has a chronic cough. He believes the cough is caused by bronchitis and stubbornly insists on being prescribed antibiotics.

Juanita Hansen is a single mother in her mid-20s with one son, Henry. Juanita arrives at the urgent care clinic for the fourth time in a month. Henry has fallen twice, suffered a burn on the hand, and is now refusing to eat.

Lenore McDonell is a disabled woman in her early 30s who lives independently, with the aid of a motorized wheelchair. Lenore functions well in her home environment but has grown fearful of venturing out, even to the physician's office for her routine follow-up examinations. She has canceled three appointments in a row.

SELF-ASSESSMENT

As you were deciding to become a medical assistant, what other careers were you considering? List the three reasons you were considering that other career, and then list three reasons you chose medical assisting instead. Keep in mind not just the time, money, and education involved, but also the profession itself, the day-to-day duties, the type of work, the people involved, and so forth.

Other career:

(1) _____

(2) _____

(3) _____

Medical assisting:

(1) _____

(2) _____

(3) _____

Think about the similarities between the two careers. Are there more similarities than differences? Are you going to be using some of the same skills? Is there a way that these two different careers will come together at any point in the future?

CHAPTER POST-TEST

This test is similar to the Pre-Test. Perform this test without looking at the book. This is just to see how well you have understood and can recall the information presented in this chapter after you have studied it and completed the workbook exercises. You will not be graded on this portion (other than the grade you give yourself), but this is an excellent preparation for your instructor's test. You may use this Post-Test to determine what areas you need to study more. Justify any "false" answers.

1. Sole proprietors work alone and do not employ other doctors. (T or F)

2. Partnerships are made up of two physicians, and corporations are made up of three or more physicians. (T or F)

3. Urgent care centers are for emergencies only. (T or F)

4. Urgent care centers require skills that medical assistants do not generally have. (T or F)

5. Managed care cannot set limits on the services your doctor provides to a patient. (T or F)

6. Physicians are licensed to practice state by state. (T or F)

7. Chiropractors only work on musculoskeletal conditions. (T or F)

8. Acupuncture can be helpful when dealing with pain and a variety of disorders in the gastro-intestinal, urogenital, gynecologic, circulatory, respiratory, neuromusculoskeletal, and many other systems. (T or F)

CERTIFICATION CRITERIA CHECK LIST

As you go through your education and training, keep in mind the national certification examination that you will take when you graduate. Each chapter of the textbook and workbook covers a different section of the examination criteria. To keep track of your preparation for the certification examination, turn to the back of this workbook and highlight the following CMA, RMA, or CMAS certification examination criteria (if you have already highlighted them from a previous chapter, put a check mark by the criteria):

CMA
A. Medical Terminology
    1. Word building and definitions
        d. Medical specialties
D. Professionalism
    5. Working as a team member to achieve goals
        a. Member responsibilities
        b. Promoting competent patient care
        c. Utilizing principles of group dynamics

RMA
I. General Medical Assisting Knowledge
    C. Medical Law
        2. Licensure, certification and registration
            a. Identify credentialing requirements of medical professionals
    E. Human Relations
        2. Interpersonal relations
            a) Employ appropriate interpersonal skills with:
                (1) Employer/Administrator
                (2) Co-Workers

CMAS
1. Medical Assisting Foundation
    • Professionalism
3. Medical Office Clerical Assisting
    • Communication

EVALUATION OF CHAPTER KNOWLEDGE

Skills	Student Self-Evaluation		
	Good	Average	Poor
I understand the concepts of managed care.	___	___	___
I have the ability to distinguish medical management models.	___	___	___
I can empathize with my patient's experiences of medical settings.	___	___	___
I have the ability to identify members of the health care team.	___	___	___
I respect professionalism.	___	___	___
I understand the medical assistant's role.	___	___	___

CHAPTER 3

History of Medicine

CHAPTER PRE-TEST

Perform this test without looking back at the textbook or the workbook. This is just to see how well you have understood and can recall the information in this chapter after you have read it, but before you have completed the workbook exercises. You will not be graded on this portion (other than the grade you give yourself). Justify any "false" answers.

1. The practice of medicine began when we started keeping medical records. (T or F)

2. Plants used to be the basis of all medications, but are not anymore. (T or F)

3. Cultural differences do not and should not influence the way we treat our patients. (T or F)

4. Magic has played a vital role in medicine. (T or F)

5. Ancient Eastern treatments included curing the spirit and nourishing the body. (T or F)

6. Acupuncture uses the placement of needles in thousands of points on the body. (T or F)

7. Women were not accepted as medical doctors in Western culture until the 1800s. (T or F)

8. The Father of Preventive Medicine was Louis Pasteur. (T or F)

9. Edward Jenner developed the smallpox vaccine in the late 1700s. (T or F)

10. The Oath of Hippocrates mentions mischief, sexual misconduct, and slaves. (T or F)

11. Medical assisting has only been around for a few years. (T or F)

INTRODUCTION

The medical assistant is a part of the constantly evolving history of medicine. Medicine developed from the contributions of individuals from various cultures throughout history who held many different theories and attitudes about medicine and the treatment of patients. Today, the advances made in medicine continue to be shaped by more than one discipline or philosophy of care and treatment. Students of medical assisting can use this workbook chapter to discover the rich history of medicine and to think about the medical assistant's role in the future of medicine and health care.

PERFORMANCE OBJECTIVES

After successful completion of this chapter you will be able to discuss the effects that culture, religion, magic, and science have had on modern medicine. You will be able to discuss common treatments used in the past and three theories or practices of ancient medicine that still are prevalent today. You will know the historical roles of specialists and women and be able to trace the progression of medical education. You will become familiar with several significant contributions to medicine, including three recent developments. *The following statements are related to your learning objectives for this chapter. Fill in the blanks with the appropriate term(s).*

Ancient Chinese beliefs states that there were several methods of treatment; they were to cure the (1) _____, nourish the (2) _____, give (3) _____, treat the whole (4) _____, and use (5) _____ and (6) _____. Many of these ancient beliefs are still excellent (7) _____ for today's health care. Religion is still an important part of health and healing. In ancient times and in some present-day cultures, certain gods were/are called on for (8) _____ through (9) _____, (10) _____, and (11) _____. Magic was used to chase away (12) _____. Common treatments used in the past were (13) _____, to cause vomiting, and (14) _____, to purge from the rectum. Women were accepted as (15) _____ in primitive societies, and later were allowed to care for (16) _____ and to assist in (17) _____. They were considered unqualified to become doctors in Western cultures until the (18) _____ century. Medical education in established universities began in the (19) _____ century. (20) _____ made anatomical preparations from which he produced drawings of the skeletal, muscular, nervous, and vascular systems. Sadly, his accurate sketch of the spinal vertebrae went undiscovered for more the (21) _____ years! We are all familiar with the Father of Bacteria, (22) _____ _____, but have you heard of (23) _____, who discovered x-rays? We certainly have come a long way since then. More recently, we are finding noninvasive methods of "looking" into the body and seeing great detail. The (24) _____, (25) _____, and (26) _____ assist in diagnosis now. Organ and tissue transplants, easy and quick laboratory tests, vaccines, and medicines are only a few of the wonderful new (27) _____ in medicine.

VOCABULARY BUILDER

Find the words below that are misspelled; circle them, and then correctly spell them in the spaces provided. Then insert the correct vocabulary terms from the list that best fit the descriptions below.

acupuncture
alopathic
asepsis
bubonic plague

malaria
moxibustion
pharmacopoeias
pluralistic

septacemia
typhis
yellow fever

_____   _____   _____

_____   _____

1. In our _____ society, we rely on several philosophies of medicine that serve an individual's needs by respecting ethnic, cultural, and religious traditions while providing the best standard of care to patients and their families.

2. _____ is an ancient Chinese technique that requires the use of a powdered plant substance that is made into a small mound on the patient's skin and then burned, usually leaving a blister.

3. The piercing of the skin by long needles into any of 365 points along 12 meridians that transverse the body and transmit an active life force called *chi* is the practice of _____, an ancient Chinese technique thought by many today to be effective in the treatment of chronic pain.

4. That bacteria can enter the bloodstream to cause infection, _____, was observed in the nineteenth century by Hungarian physician and obstetrician Ignaz Philipp Semmelweis. He proved that physicians who came from an autopsy directly to the care of postpartum women, without scrubbing their hands and washing instruments, carried infection with them that often caused puerperal fever and death in new mothers.

5. In the twentieth century, the discovery of antibiotics, the development of vaccines, and the institution of proper health and sanitation measures have largely contributed to the containment of many infectious diseases, including _____, _____, and _____. However, new drug-resistant strains of tuberculosis, _____, and other diseases are not responding to known treatments, presenting medical researchers with new challenges for the twenty-first century.

6. Homeopathic physicians treat illness and disease by nonsurgical methods using small doses of medicine, based on the theory that "like cures like." _____ physicians treat illness and disease with medical and surgical interventions intended to alleviate the condition or effect a cure.

7. World cultures throughout history have compiled unique_____: books describing drugs and their preparation that detail plant, animal, and mineral substances as essential ingredients in effecting cures.

8. In the nineteenth century, _____, the process of sterilizing surgical environments to discourage the growth of bacteria, and anesthesia, the process of alleviating pain during surgery, revolutionized surgical practices throughout the world.

LEARNING REVIEW

1. A. Religion, magic, and science all play a vital part in the history of medicine. Why?

Religion_____

_____

_____

Magic_____

_____

_____

Science _____

_____

_____

B. *For each of the following, write an R if belief in religion, an M if belief in magic, or an S if belief in science underlies the treatment or practice.*

_____ 1. A recent research study involved two groups of patients with AIDS: one group received daily prayers from an anonymous prayer group hundreds of miles away, and the other received no prayers. The group receiving the prayers responded better to treatment.

_____ 2. Trephination was used by prehistoric cultures to release evil spirits responsible for illness.

_____ 3. Chinese acupuncture techniques are used to control pain or treat drug dependency.

_____ 4. Botanicals are effective in treating certain conditions. The Chinese pharmacopoeia is rich in the use of herbs.

_____ 5. Some Native Americans believe that someone recovering from a serious illness might hold extraordinary powers.

_____ 6. Some physicians throughout history have held to the belief that healing involves not just medical treatment, but attention to the purity of the patient's soul and an attention to the faith of the individual as well.

2. Name the five methods of treatment important to the practice of medicine according to ancient Chinese tradition. How are these methods relevant for allopathic physicians today?

(1) _____

_____

(2) _____

_____

(3) _____

_____

(4) _____

_____

(5) _____

_____

3. Individual cultures and people throughout history have conferred different, and often changing, status to women in medicine. For each of the five cultures below, describe the status of women in medicine.

Primitive societies _____

_____

_____

_____

Chinese _____

_____

_____

_____

Muslim _____

_____

_____

_____

Italian _____

_____

_____

_____

American _____

_____

_____

_____

4. Trace the progression of medical education by listing the important advances, discoveries, or medical philosophies for each period or century listed. What do you expect for the twenty-first century?

Prehistoric times _____

_____

_____

_____

_____

Ancient times _____

_____

_____

_____

Seventh century _____

_____

_____

_____

Ninth century _____

_____

_____

_____

Renaissance _____

_____

_____

_____

Nineteenth century _____

_____

_____

_____

Twentieth century _____

_____

_____

_____

_____

_____

Twenty-first century_____

_____

_____

_____

_____

5. Attitudes toward illness have changed throughout the history of medicine and also often differ between cultures. For each situation listed, give both historical and current attitudes toward the sick person. Discuss how attitudes toward illness may, or may not, have changed through history.

A. Elderly and infirm people are encouraged to end their own lives or are outcast from society.

_____

_____

_____

B. Individuals with a frightening illness, for which there is no cure, are shunned or quarantined.

_____

_____

_____

C. Sickness is seen as a moral or spiritual failing of an individual.

_____

_____

_____

D. Survivors of illness are viewed as heroic individuals.

_____

_____

_____

E. People with disabilities are valued as individuals and receive care that allows them to function in mainstream society.

_____

_____

_____

6. Name 12 infectious or epidemic diseases that have been controlled in the twentieth century through medical advances and discoveries such as antibiotics, vaccines, asepsis, and insulin.

(1) _____   (6) _____   (11) _____

(2) _____   (7) _____   (12) _____

(3) _____   (8) _____

(4) _____   (9) _____

(5) _____   (10) _____

7. The Hippocratic Oath, which originated in ancient Greece, embodied within it many ethical standards of treatment and care that physicians espouse even today. List, in contemporary layperson's language, the five basic standards contained in the oath.

(1) _____

(2) _____

(3) _____

(4) _____

(5) _____

8. *Match each individual with their contribution to the history of medicine. In the space following each name, fill in the century in which the individual lived.*

____ 1. Andreas Vesalius _____   A. developed a vaccine for poliomyelitis
____ 2. Sir Alexander Fleming _____   B. Father of Medicine
____ 3. W. T. G. Morton _____   C. developed smallpox vaccine
____ 4. Moses _____   D. discovered penicillin
____ 5. Edward Jenner _____   E. Father of Bacteriology
____ 6. Clara Barton _____   F. advocate of health rules in Hebrew
____ 7. Louis Pasteur _____   religion
____ 8. Elizabeth Blackwell _____   G. invented the stethoscope
____ 9. Hippocrates _____   H. first female physician in the United
____ 10. René Laënnec _____   States
____ 11. Robert Koch _____   I. rendered accurate anatomical
____ 12. Florence Nightingale _____   drawings of body systems
____ 13. Anton van Leeuwenhoek _____   J. wrote first anatomical studies
____ 14. Wilhelm Roetgen _____   K. laid the groundwork on asepsis
____ 15. John Hunter _____   L. started the American Red Cross
____ 16. Elizabeth G. Anderson _____   M. founder of modern nursing
____ 17. Leonardo da Vinci _____   N. introduced ether as anesthetic
____ 18. Joseph Lister _____   O. discovered lens magnification
____ 19. Jonas Salk _____   P. discovered x rays
____ 20. Frederick G. Banting _____   Q. founder of scientific surgery
                                           R. developed culture-plate method
                                           S. discovered insulin
                                           T. first female physician in Britain

9. The ancient culture that believed that illness was a punishment by the gods for violations of moral codes was the:
   a. Chinese
   b. Egyptian
   c. Mesopotamian
   d. Indian

10. Ancient healing priests performed many functions that involved the welfare of the entire community or village and were referred to as:
    a. shaman
    b. chi
    c. lipuria
    d. polypenia

11. Medical education in established universities began in what century?
    a. second
    b. fifteenth
    c. eighteenth
    d. ninth

12. What country today quarantines everyone who tests positive for HIV, even if they show no signs of the disease?
    a. Africa
    b. Cuba
    c. Korea
    d. Canada

13. In 1922, insulin was founded as a treatment for diabetes by:
    a. Lister
    b. Pasteur
    c. Salk and Sabin
    d. Banting and Best

CERTIFICATION REVIEW

These questions are designed to mimic the certification examinations. You can use these questions like a small "Certification Examination Study Guide," but this is not meant to take the place of the more extensive study guides. Use this portion to determine in what areas to concentrate your efforts when studying for the certification examination.

1. Who of the following was not a scientist who contributed to the study of bacteriology?
   a. Louis Pasteur
   b. Robert Koch
   c. Joseph Lister
   d. John Hunter

2. The first female physician in the United States was:
   a. Clara Barton
   b. Elizabeth Blackwell
   c. Florence Nightingale
   d. Joan of Arc

3. The Oath of Hippocrates:
   a. establishes guidelines for all health care providers
   b. establishes guidelines for the practice of medicine
   c. is a well-known document about the ethics of ancient medicine
   d. was the first scientific journal of significance

CASE STUDY

When 52-year-old Margaret Thomas, Martin Gordon's younger sister, begins to experience mild hand tremors and balance problems, Martin suggests that Margaret go see Dr. Winston Lewis, Martin's primary care physician assisting in the treatment of his prostate cancer. Feeling more comfortable with a female physician, Margaret chooses to make an appointment with Dr. Lewis's associate in the group practice, Dr. Elizabeth King. On the day of the examination, she brings her 25-year-old daughter with her to the physician's office.

After taking a detailed patient history and undertaking a thorough physical examination of Margaret Thomas, Dr. King makes note of signs and symptoms, including a resting tremor, shuffling gait, muscle rigidity, and difficulty in swallowing and speaking. Margaret also complains of a "hot feeling" and odd, uncharacteristic moments of defective judgment when "she just can't keep things straight." Dr. King suspects Parkinson's disease and tells Margaret and her daughter that she'd like to refer Margaret to a neurologist for more specific examination and medical tests. Dr. King explains that there are effective drug therapies for controlling the disease, although it has no known cure, and that the neurologist will outline Margaret's treatment options if a diagnosis of Parkinson's is made. Margaret seems to be shaken but takes Dr. King's words in stride.

Dr. King leaves Margaret and her daughter in the examination room with Audrey Jones, C.M.A., who has assisted Dr. King throughout the examination and asks Audrey to be sure to give Mrs. Thomas the referral to the neurologist. Margaret's daughter asks Audrey if Parkinson's is the disease that has shown promise in fetal tissue research, and if her mother might be a candidate. Before Audrey can answer, Margaret becomes visibly distressed. "We're a good Catholic family, I could never consider that. Me, a grandmother." Looking to Audrey, she adds, "Please tell me I won't be involved with such a thing."

Discuss the following:
1. What part does the role of women in medicine and in society play in this situation?
2. How should medical assistant Audrey Jones reply to Mrs. Thomas and her daughter? What course of action, if any, should she take?
3. How do religious beliefs make an impact on the attitude toward illness held by the patient? How might these beliefs affect a treatment plan?
4. Discuss the issues that arise when a potential medical breakthrough involves controversial or radical ideas that challenge long-held cultural viewpoints and beliefs.

SELF-ASSESSMENT

A. Make a list of the various ethnic, religious, and cultural groups you and your family members participate in or are descended from.

B. Interview family members to determine how their ethnic, religious, or cultural beliefs make an impact on the kind of medical care and treatment they expect to receive and how attitudes may have changed or evolved from generation to generation. Write a brief summary of your family's beliefs.

C. Write down any folk or home remedies used by your parents or grandparents that may or may not still be used by your family today. Why might these remedies have been more widely relied on by previous generations? Is there a scientific basis for each remedy?

CHAPTER POST-TEST

This is similar to your Pre-Test. Perform this test without looking at the book. This is just to see how well you have understood and can recall the information presented in this chapter after you have studied it and completed the workbook exercises. You will not be graded on this portion (other than the grade you give yourself), but this is an excellent preparation for your instructor's test. You may use this Post-Test to determine what areas you need to study more. Justify any "false" answers.

1. The practice of medicine began long before we started keeping medical records. (T or F)

2. Plants remain the basis of many medications. (T or F)

3. Cultural differences do and should influence the way we treat our patients. (T or F)

4. Magic has never played a vital role in medicine. (T or F)

5. Ancient Eastern treatments did not include working with the human spirit. (T or F)

6. Acupuncture uses the placement of needles in 365 points on the body. (T or F)

7. Women were accepted as medical doctors in Chinese culture long before Western cultures. (T or F)

8. The Father of Preventive Medicine was Joseph Lister. (T or F)

9. Edward Jenner developed the smallpox vaccine in the late 1800s. (T or F)

EVALUATION OF CHAPTER KNOWLEDGE

Skills	Student Self-Evaluation		
	Good	Average	Poor
I am sensitive to cultural, ethnic, and religious beliefs of others.	_____	_____	_____
I understand the importance of mutual respect in the physician–patient relationship.	_____	_____	_____
I have the ability to identify attitudes toward illness.	_____	_____	_____
I have the ability to trace major discoveries and contributions to history of medicine.	_____	_____	_____
I recognize major figures of medical history.	_____	_____	_____
I show patience and open-mindedness toward others.	_____	_____	_____
I have the ability to describe the role of the medical assistant in the future of medicine.	_____	_____	_____

CHAPTER 4

Therapeutic Communication Skills

CHAPTER PRE-TEST

Perform this test without looking at the book. This is just to see how well you have understood and can recall the information in this chapter after you have read it, but before you have completed the workbook exercises. You will not be graded on this portion (other than the grade you give yourself). Justify any "false" answers.

1. Gestures and expressions have nothing to do with what a person is thinking or feeling. (T or F)
2. You can make sick patients "feel better" just by the way you communicate with them. (T or F)
3. Everyone enjoys a hug. (T or F)
4. While speaking on the phone a patient can tell how you are feeling. (T or F)

INTRODUCTION

The word *therapeutic* basically means "to aid in health" or to "make better." Therapeutic communication implies that the interaction (verbal or nonverbal) between you, as the medical assistant, and your patients should help them heal or at least should make them feel better. And, studies show, when we feel better, we are healthier. If we extend the therapeutic communication to our coworkers, our physician–employers, and into our personal lives, we all benefit.

Now all we have to agree on is: What makes up therapeutic communication? Some people enjoy a more intimate interaction, perhaps a touch on the arm, whereas others prefer a more distant, formal interaction. Some of these preferences come from our families and how we were raised, some are cultural, and some are developed through our personal experiences. However we obtain our personal preferences on how we like to be treated, we can all probably agree that a caring, professional manner is always appreciated. The traditional Golden Rule says: "Do unto others as you would have them do unto you"; in essence, treat people how you would like to be treated. The new Golden Rule says: "Treat others as they want to be treated." To abide by the new Golden Rule, we must understand other people; that is, where they come from, their culture, their heritage, and their attitudes toward health care.

Use this workbook chapter to explore the many components of effective therapeutic communication, cultivate the ability to learn and observe, recognize and respond to messages communicated both verbally and nonverbally, consider patients' needs with empathy and impartiality, and adapt your communication to meet the receivers' abilities to understand. In personal, face-to-face communication, as well as in telephone conversations, the medical assistant's goal is to achieve a level of therapeutic communication that enhances the patient's comfort level and eases the pathway of communication between the patient and the health care team.

PERFORMANCE OBJECTIVES

After successful completion of this chapter, you should be able to explain what therapeutic means, to differentiate between verbal and nonverbal communication, and be aware of your own communication style. You should have learned how to communicate with your patients, family, coworkers, and supervisors using effective and professional communication skills. Try not to look back at the introductory section of this workbook chapter as you fill in the blanks in the following paragraph. If necessary, reread the Introduction. *The following statements are related to your learning objectives for this chapter. Fill in the blanks with the appropriate term(s):*

The word *therapeutic* basically means (1) _____ or to

(2) _____. Therapeutic (3) _____ can be either

(4) _____ or (5) _____, but it should always help your patient

(6) _____. Therapeutic communication should also encompass your

(7) _____, (8) _____, and (9) _____.

Our communication preferences come from (10) _____,

(11) _____, our (12) _____ and even

(13) _____. Most people prefer a (14) _____

and (15) _____ manner, though. The new Golden Rule says:

(16) _____. To honor this method

of treating people, we must understand (17)_____,

(18) _____, (19) _____,

and (20) _____. This chapter will help

you explore therapeutic communication and (21) _____,

(22) _____,

(23) _____ and

(24) _____.

VOCABULARY BUILDER

Find the words below that are misspelled; circle them, and then correctly spell them in the spaces provided. Then insert the correct vocabulary terms from the list that best fit the descriptions below.

active listening
biases
body language
buffer words
closed questions
cluster
congruancy

decode
encode
hierarcky of needs
indirect statements
interview technigues
kinesics
masking

open-ended questions
perseption
prejudices
roadblocks to communication
therapuetic communication

_____   _____   _____

_____   _____

1. _____ Communication that allows patients to feel comfortable, even when receiving difficult or unpleasant information, achieved through use of specific and well-defined professional communication skills.

2. The italicized words in the following statement are examples of: _____. "*Good afternoon, this is* Inner City Health Care. *This is* Walter Seals. How may I help you?"

3. _____ Adept use of these methods encourages the best communication between health care professionals and patients, equalizing the relationship as much as possible.

4. _____ The specific order or rank within which a person's needs are met, moving from the most basic needs to self-actualization.

5. _____ These types of questions require only a yes or no answer: "Mrs. Leonard, are you feeling dizzy now?"

6. _____ These potential verbal or nonverbal messages that prevent a successful cycle of communication can be overcome by the medical assistant's sensitivity to patients' personalities and needs.

7. _____ The study of body language explores methods of nonverbal communication that accompany speech.

8. _____ These statements turn a question into a topic of interest that allows the patient to speak without feeling directly questioned: "Mr. Taylor, tell me about any difficulties your father's dementia presents with daily living activities at home."

9. _____ As Marilyn Johnson takes his family history for the patient record, Jim Marshall says repeatedly, "I am worried because my father died from a heart attack at a young age." Marilyn uses this kind of therapeutic communication to rephrase the message by responding, "You are concerned about your cardiovascular health and your genetic risk?"

10. _____ These personal preferences denote a predisposition for one particular belief or viewpoint over another.

11. _____ These beliefs or viewpoints represent preconceived notions an individual may have formed before all the facts are known.

12. _____ John O'Keefe sat with a sullen expression, eyes downcast, his arms folded across his chest, as he spoke to medical assistant Joe Guerrero about the financial hardships his family would face if his wife, Mary, were pregnant again. Joe relies on Mr. O'Keefe's nonverbal communication to convey his repressed feelings of anger.

13. _____ These types of questions require more than a yes or no answer: "Ms. Johnson, how are you doing with the special diet Dr. Lewis suggested?"

14. _____ This attempt to hide from or repress obscures one's true feelings or real message.

15. _____ Nonverbal messages grouped together to form, in aggregate, a statement or conclusion.

16. _____ Medical assistant Karen Ritter nods her head yes as she explains to Annette Samuels that insurance will cover any medical tests related to her stomach cramps. Karen's nonverbal message agrees with her verbal message.

17. _____ The receiver must interpret the meaning of the message to understand it.

18. _____ The sender creates a message carefully crafted to match the receiver's ability to receive and interpret it properly.

19. _____ This kind of intuitive realization involves an active understanding of one's own feelings *and* the feelings of others.

Crossword Puzzle

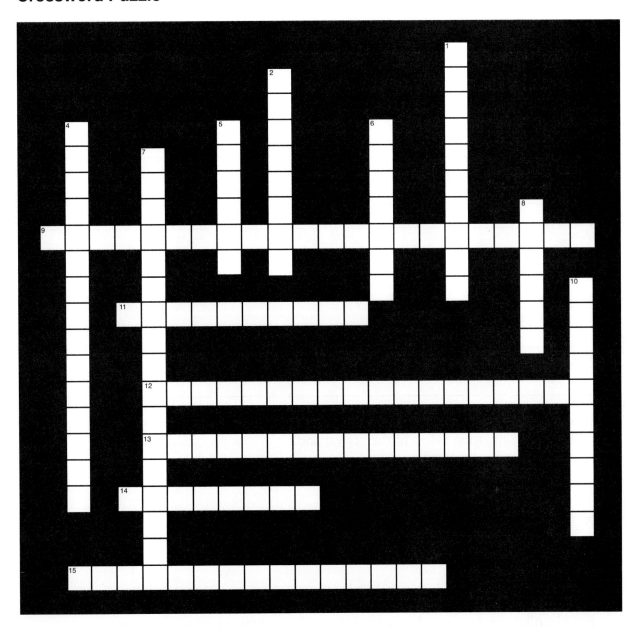

Across

9. Gestures and expressions together with body poses
11. Moving back to a former stage to escape conflict
12. Involves sending and receiving messages, verbal and nonverbal
13. The art of really hearing another person's message and sometimes verifying with them what you are hearing
14. The study of body movements
15. Questions that can be answered with a simple yes or no

Down

1. An opinion or judgement that is formed before all the facts are known
2. Giving the speaker information about what you are hearing
4. The act of justification, usually illogically, that people use to keep from facing the truth
5. The rejection or refusal to acknowledge information
6. The position of the body and parts of the body
7. Behavior that protects people from feelings of guilt, anxiety, and shame
8. A slant toward a particular belief
10. Sometimes referred to as temporary amnesia

LEARNING REVIEW

1. Culture presents a profound influence on successful therapeutic communication. For the seven cultural influences that follow, list one way in which each of them makes an impact on therapeutic communication.

   Ethnic heritage _____

   _____

   Geographic location and background _____

   _____

   Genetics_____

   _____

   Economics _____

   _____

   Educational experiences _____

   _____

   Life experiences _____

   _____

   Personal value systems_____

   _____

2. Biases and prejudices common in today's society have the potential to create hostility. Match each difficult situation below to the corresponding bias or prejudice that motivates it. Put a letter in the space provided.

   A. A preference for Western-style medicine.

   B. The tendency to choose female rather than male physicians.

   C. Prejudice related to a person's sexual preference.

   D. Discrimination based on race or religion.

   E. Hostile attitudes toward persons with a value system opposite your own.

   F. A belief that persons who cannot afford health care should receive less care than someone who can pay for full services.

   _____ 1. Mr. Gordon refuses to accept a referral to an acupuncturist to help alleviate the chronic pain of advancing prostate cancer.

   _____ 2. Medical assistant Bruce Goldman mistakenly assumes that patient Bill Schwartz has AIDS when he arrives at the clinic with a gentleman friend, seeking attention for a recurring black mole on this calf.

   _____ 3. Rhoda and Lee Au fear they will not receive adequate medical care because they use Chinese as their first language and speak only broken English.

_____ 4. Corey Boyer resists his gym teacher's efforts to get him to the clinic to check out a recurring rash on his arm because his family has no health insurance.

_____ 5. Mary O'Keefe is relieved to find that the practice's OB/GYN is a female physician, Dr. Elizabeth King.

_____ 6. Edith Leonard, a widow in her 70s, counsels medical assistant Liz Corbin that she should settle down and get married instead of pursuing a dream to attend medical school and become a pediatrician.

3. The four modes of communication most pertinent in our everyday exchange are:

(1) _____   (3) _____

(2) _____   (4) _____

4. Active listening is an important element of therapeutic communication. To practice active listening skills, rephrase each of the messages listed for verification from the sender; also include a therapeutic response.

A. "I don't know what to do. My father takes so many pills he can't remember which is the right one, so he ends up refusing to take any of them."

_____

_____

_____

B. "I can't give you my insurance card; I lost it, and I don't remember the name of the company either. But you've always taken care of it before."

_____

_____

_____

C. "I can't help being worried. The doctor just suggested a referral for treatment at that hospital where somebody had their wrong foot operated on. What do you think?"

_____

_____

_____

D. "I feel dizzy just thinking about having my blood taken. Do you really need to do it?"

_____

_____

_____

5. *Circle the five correct responses.*

The five Cs of communication are:

clear	complete	courteous
coherent	concise	credible
cohesive	constant	curious
comment	cooperative	curt

6. Abraham Maslow, the founder of humanistic psychology, postulated that a person's needs move from the most basic of survival to the state of self-actualization. Self-actualization occurs when the person realizes the maximum of human potential. Each level of need must be met before an individual can proceed successfully to the next level. Understanding Maslow's hierarchy will help medical assistants assess patients' needs and facilitate therapeutic communication. For each level, list a minimum of three needs that meet it.

   Survival or physiological needs _____

   _____

   _____

   Safety needs _____

   _____

   Belongingness and love needs _____

   _____

   _____

   Prestige and esteem needs _____

   _____

   _____

7. Identify eight significant roadblocks to communication.

   (1) _____   (5) _____

   (2) _____   (6) _____

   (3) _____   (7) _____

   (4) _____   (8) _____

8. Edith Leonard arrives at the clinic for a routine 6-month follow-up examination. At her last visit, she had been referred to an ophthalmologist for removal of a cataract in her right eye. Compose a closed question, open-ended question, and indirect statement regarding Ms. Leonard's condition.

   Closed question _____

   _____

   Open-ended question _____

   _____

   Indirect statement _____

   _____

9. Telephone communication between medical assistants and patients is an important kind of therapeutic communication. Tone and pace of voice, together with word choice, carry the message when there is no visual feedback. List four tools of communication essential to conducting successful telephone conversations.

   (1) _____

   _____

   (2) _____

   _____

   (3) _____

   _____

   (4) _____

   _____

10. The conscious awareness of one's own feelings and the feelings of others is:

    a. congruency

    b. perception

    c. bias

    d. masking

11. The founder of humanistic psychology is:

    a. Jacobi

    b. Freud

    c. Erikson

    d. Maslow

12. The lifeline of the physician's office is:

    a. the facsimile machine

    b. telecommunication conferencing

    c. the telephone

    d. e-mail

13. The grouping of nonverbal messages into statements or conclusions is known as:

    a. assimilating

    b. feedback

    c. clustering

    d. introjection

CERTIFICATION REVIEW

These questions are designed to mimic the certification examinations. You can use these questions like a small "Certification Examination Study Guide," but this is not meant to take the place of the more extensive study guides. Use this portion to determine where to concentrate your efforts when studying for the certification examination.

1. Which of the following is not part of communication?
   a. speech
   b. facial expression
   c. gestures
   d. attitude
   e. body positioning

2. Which is the most basic of Maslow's hierarchy of needs?
   a. food
   b. safety
   c. status and self-esteem
   d. need for knowledge
   e. self-actualization

3. Your patient refuses to accept a diagnosis, claiming the doctor "must be mistaken." Assuming the doctor is correct, which self-defense mechanism is the patient using?
   a. repression
   b. denial
   c. projection
   d. compensation
   e. rationalization

4. Congruency in communication can be described as:
   a. when the verbal message matches the facial expression
   b. when the verbal message does not match the gestures
   c. when the verbal message can be interpreted in two or more different ways
   d. when two different messages are interpreted as the same

CASE STUDY

Wayne Elder arrives at the clinic for an examination to check on a recurrent ear infection that has been treated with antibiotics. Wayne, who is slightly retarded and lives in a group home, is still reporting dizziness and pain in his ear. He has come to the clinic by himself, taking a bus from his job as a part-time dishwasher. Wayne's boss asked him to return to the clinic because Wayne could not concentrate at work.

Clinical medical assistant Wanda Slawson discovers from Wayne that he has not been taking his medication properly; he stopped taking pills once his ear began to feel better. She must politely ask Wayne to repeat himself several times before she can clearly understand his slurred speech, and she has difficulty holding his attention or maintaining eye contact.

Wanda conveys Wayne's situation to Dr. Ray Reynolds, who examines Wayne and gives him a new prescription for antibiotics, gently explaining the need to finish the entire prescription to get well. After Dr. Reynolds leaves the examination room, however, it is clear to Wanda that Wayne is still confused about why he must take the medication even after he begins to feel better. Wanda carefully explains to Wayne that the infection will continue to heal even though he no longer feels sick. To be sure he understands, Wanda asks Wayne to repeat to her what he must do and why; she then asks Dr. Reynolds to step in briefly to remind Wayne once more to complete the prescription.

Discuss the following issues:
1. How does the unequal relationship that exists between patients and health care professionals have an impact on the therapeutic communication between physician, medical assistant, and patient?
2. How must medical assistant Wanda Slawson tailor her verbal and nonverbal messages to meet the abilities of her receivers: the physician (Dr. Ray Reynolds) and the patient (Wayne Elder)?
3. How does Wanda use active listening? Which interview techniques are the most effective in facilitating therapeutic communication? Does nonverbal communication play a role?
4. Using Maslow's hierarchy of needs, discuss how the health care team meets Wayne's special needs resulting from his disability.
5. Do you think the medical assistant acted appropriately? What else could she have done? What should she not do in this situation?

SELF-ASSESSMENT

Think about your own facial expressions and body language. Are you always portraying the message you want to send? List two situations in which you have been misinterpreted through your nonverbal communication, or situations in which you have misinterpreted someone else's message. Then think of what would have been a verbal message to help make the situation more accurate. That is, explain what you could have said to the person to determine if he or she was really hearing the message you meant to send.

(1) _____

_____

_____

(2) _____

_____

_____

CHAPTER POST-TEST

This is similar to the Pre-Test. Perform this test without looking at the book. This is just to see how well you have understood and can recall the information presented in this chapter after you have studied it and completed the workbook exercises. You will not be graded on this portion (other than the grade you give yourself), but this is an excellent preparation for your instructor's test. You may use this Post-Test to determine what areas you need to study more. Justify any "false" answers.

1. Gestures and expressions can always tell you what a person is thinking or feeling. (T or F)
2. You can make a sick patient "feel worse" just by the way you communicate with them. (T or F)
3. Hugs are universally acceptable as a means of communicating. (T or F)
4. While speaking on the phone you can tell how a patient is feeling. (T or F)

CERTIFICATION CRITERIA CHECKLIST

As you go through your education and training, keep in mind the national certification examination that you will take when you graduate. Each chapter of the textbook and workbook covers a different section of the examination criteria. To keep track of your preparation for the certification examination, turn to the back of this workbook and highlight the following CMA, RMA, or CMAS certification examination criteria (if you have already highlighted them from a previous chapter, put a check mark by the criteria):

CMA
C. Psychology
     1. Basic principles
     3. Hereditary, cultural and environmental influences on behavior
     4. Defense mechanisms
E. Communication
     2. Recognizing and responding to verbal and nonverbal communication
     4. Professional communication and behavior
          a. Professional situations
          b. Therapeutic relationships
     5. Evaluating and understanding communication

RMA
I. General Medical Assisting Knowledge
     E. Human Relations
          1. Patient relations
          2. Interpersonal relations

CMAS
1. Medical Assisting Foundation
     • Professionalism
3. Medical Office Clerical Assisting
     • Communication

COMPETENCY ASSESSMENT
Procedure 4-1 Identifying Community Resources

Performance Objectives: To have a list of community resources available for patient use. Perform this objective within 30 minutes with a minimum score of 20 points.

Supplies/Equipment: Computer and printer, multiple resources from a variety of community services.

Charting/Documentation: Enter appropriate documentation/charting in the box.

_____

_____

_____

Instructor's/Evaluator's Comments and Suggestions:

_____

_____

_____

_____

SKILLS CHECKLIST Procedure 4-1: Identify Community Resources

Name _____

Date _____

No.	Skill	Check #1 20 pts ea	Check #2 10 pts ea	Check #3 5 pts ea	Notes
1	Determine the type of information to be in your data base.				
2	Contact the sources and request any listings they may have.				
3	Search the Internet to obtain the desired resources.				
4	Develop a database on your computer so you can search easily for the resource when needed. Maintain a notebook with the resource information printed and indexed.				
Student's Total Points					
Points Possible		80	40	20	
Final Score (Student's Total Points / Possible Points)					
		Notes			
Start time:					
End time:					
Total time: (30 min goal)					

EVALUATION OF CHAPTER KNOWLEDGE

Skills	Student Self-Evaluation		
	Good	Average	Poor
I can identify my personal communication strengths.	____	____	____
I can indentify areas for improvement in my personal communication style.	____	____	____
I listen well.	____	____	____
I cultivate sharp observation skills.	____	____	____
I recognize and respond to verbal and nonverbal communication.	____	____	____
I understand the communication cycle.	____	____	____
I can adapt my communication to individuals' abilities to understand.	____	____	____
I consider patients' needs with empathy and impartiality.	____	____	____
I have the ability to identify roadblocks to communication and defense mechanisms.	____	____	____
I know how to use proper telephone technique.	____	____	____
I practice successful therapeutic communication.	____	____	____

CHAPTER 5

Coping Skills for the Medical Assistant

CHAPTER PRE-TEST

Perform this test without looking at the book. This is just to see how well you have understood and can recall the information in this chapter after you have read it, but before you have completed the workbook exercises. You will not be graded on this portion (other than the grade you give yourself). Justify any "false" answers.

1. Stress is always something bad. (T or F)

2. Stress is something we cannot prevent. (T or F)

3. If you have a lot of responsibility in your job, you cannot avoid burnout. (T or F)

4. Setting goals helps relieve stress (T or F)

INTRODUCTION

Medical assistants and other health care professionals occasionally feel the stress of working in the demanding and challenging field of medicine and health care. Health care professionals must maintain a high level of skill and proficiency and possess knowledge about new technologies and medical advances. Whether juggling a full patient schedule, facing difficult—and sometimes life-or-death—situations with patients, or balancing administrative duties with a constant flow of paperwork, medical assistants take part in every phase of patient care. Students learning about medical assisting can use this workbook chapter to learn about handling stress in the workplace environment of the ambulatory care setting; discover how the body adapts to stress and how to use techniques for coping with stress and avoiding burnout; and consider possible short- and long-range career goals that can act as a centering and motivating influence, further reducing stress and increasing confidence.

PERFORMANCE OBJECTIVES

After successful completion of this chapter you will understand what stress is and how you can control your personal reactions to stressors. You will recognize the stages leading up to burnout and how to avoid burnout. You will also be able to set goals, both short and long range, at work and in your personal life. Try not to look back at the textbook as you fill in the blanks in the following paragraph. If necessary, reread the textbook chapter. *The following statements are related to your learning objectives for this chapter. Fill in the blanks with the appropriate term(s):*

Medical assistants are likely to feel the (1) _____ of stress from time to time, even in the most (2) _____ _____ ambulatory care settings. We need to learn how to (3) _____ stress and handle (4) _____ in both our everyday personal lives and in our (5) _____. One of the ways to decrease stress is to recognize our personal (6) _____ so that we can gain control over our reactions to them. Another way to gain control is to set (7) _____, both (8) _____ range and (9) _____ range. The research shows that if we don't have control over our lives, (10) _____ _____ _____. Stress and frustration can lead to (11) _____. The four stages leading to this damaging state are: (12) _____, (13) _____, (14) _____, and (15) _____. If we learn to (16) _____ these stages, we can regain (17) _____ over our situations and take steps to make (18) _____.

VOCABULARY BUILDER

Find the words below that are misspelled; circle them, and then correctly spell them in the spaces provided. Then insert the correct letter of the vocabulary terms from the list that best fits the descriptions below.

A. burnout
B. goal
C. inter-directed people

D. long-range goals
E. outer-directed people
F. self-actuazation

G. short-range goals
H. stress
I. stressers

_____   _____   _____

1.____ James Whitney is a physician at Inner City Health Care. He hopes to go into private practice after gaining a few more years' experience at the urgent care center where he now works. James eventually would like to practice family medicine.

2.____ Mark Woo, another physician at Inner City Health Care, prefers emergency medicine and often pulls double shifts working with emergency patients. Although he loves the work, Mark is experiencing chronic fatigue, frequently becomes angry at coworkers, and is prone to sudden and explosive displays of emotion.

3.____ Ellen Armstrong, CMA, is usually a calming influence in the offices of Drs. Lewis and King. Lately, however, it seems to Ellen that circumstances beyond her control are threatening to pull her down. An influx of new patients into the group practice has Ellen continually backed up with filing and paperwork, her steady baby-sitter announced she'll be unavailable for the summer months, and today her car broke down on the way to work.

4.____ When Dr. Mark Woo tells emergency patient Annette Samuels that her severe stomach cramps may be caused by problems with her ovaries or appendix, she begins to feel panicky. Annette's blood pressure goes up, her breathing becomes rapid as her pulse quickens, and her eyes grow wide.

5.____ Audrey Jones, CMA, enrolls at a local college for a night-school biology class as a first step toward her goal of obtaining a bachelor's degree.

6.____ Dr. Elizabeth King, now in her mid-30s, always knew what she wanted to do with her life. After graduating from Kansas University and Stanford University Medical School, Beth searched for a physician with whom to begin a group practice and found the perfect partner in Winston Lewis.

7.____ Marilyn Johnson, CMA, office manager at the offices of Lewis and King, MD, enjoys her work and her life. Her children are grown and successful. With a master's degree in education, Marilyn teaches part-time at a local community college and is active in her town's music and art circles. She is a past president of the local chapter of the AAMA. Marilyn has worked hard to achieve the full potential of her abilities and talents and is now reaping the benefits of effort well spent.

8.____ Maria Jover takes what life gives her, deeply believing that she has no power to change her circumstances or take charge of her life. Now, Dr. King says her chronic fatigue and gynecology problems may be symptoms of AIDS, contracted from a blood transfusion she received after a severe car accident that happened several years ago. "This horrible disease will take over my life," Maria tells Dr. King.

9.____ Leo McKay is an elderly Irish Catholic man who has been laid off from his manufacturing job of 20 years. Leo asks easygoing Bruce Goldman, CMA, as he prepares Leo for a routine physical examination, "Do you have something you're working toward, some ambition for yourself—big or small?"

Word Search

Find the words in the grid below. They may go in any direction. When you are finished, the first few unused letters will form a hidden message.

```
T  A  K  E  C  A  R  E  O  F  Y  O  U  R  N  S  E  L  E  F
S  R  O  S  S  E  R  T  S  X  K  L  E  G  O  J  D  M  L  Y
L  L  J  C  K  L  K  K  C  Y  F  L  G  M  I  E  X  R  P  T
T  R  T  F  O  L  F  J  R  G  O  P  W  J  T  X  D  R  O  B
K  H  T  P  H  P  S  G  M  R  T  X  E  Z  A  H  R  S  E  H
L  W  G  R  R  T  I  X  X  Y  N  M  J  M  T  A  F  H  P  H
T  T  F  I  R  I  F  N  T  R  I  G  L  J  P  U  H  O  D  S
H  G  C  E  L  C  O  U  G  T  F  M  L  T  A  S  L  R  E  L
R  R  S  I  R  F  O  R  G  S  F  F  Z  X  D  T  B  T  T  A
M  S  R  R  L  N  R  N  I  R  K  J  K  D  A  I  M  R  C  O
N  C  B  M  R  F  I  O  U  T  L  I  Q  R  T  O  K  A  E  G
N  G  T  U  X  G  N  S  T  Q  I  X  L  L  Y  N  P  N  R  E
Y  Q  B  V  A  C  T  O  R  H  R  Z  H  L  K  Q  Z  G  I  G
T  W  J  N  D  R  Z  C  C  P  G  L  I  Z  S  M  Z  E  D  N
C  R  A  J  A  H  F  F  Z  E  R  I  Z  N  T  H  K  G  R  A
W  M  T  T  J  G  D  V  T  V  L  Q  F  T  G  B  Y  O  E  R
H  Y  I  C  O  N  T  R  O  L  T  O  T  H  N  M  R  A  N  G
Z  O  R  R  S  L  A  O  G  Q  N  T  R  C  M  P  T  L  N  N
N  Z  R  T  J  Z  K  H  N  L  C  V  K  Y  N  M  V  S  I  O
O  U  T  E  R  D  I  R  E  C  T  E  D  P  E  O  P  L  E  L
```

adaptation	long-range goals
burnout	managing time
control	outer-directed people
coping skills	prioritizing
exhaustion	role
fight or flight	role conflict
frustration	short-range goals
goals	stress
inner-directed people	stressors

LEARNING REVIEW

1. Han Selye's general adaptation syndrome (GAS) theory proposes that adaptation to stress occurs in four stages. Identify each stage in the order in which it is manifested and describe the physiologic changes that occur during each stage.

    (1) _____

    _____

    _____

    (2) _____

    _____

    _____

    (3) _____

    _____

    _____

    (4) _____

    _____

    _____

2. Match each of the following activities to its correct approach for coping with stress in the workplace.

    A. Plan ahead
    B. Arrive early
    C. Managing your lifestyle
    D. Laugh
    E. Music/Color/Light
    F. Breaks
    G. Work smarter, not harder

    _____ 1. Soothe and promote relaxation by softly playing a calming classical CD in the reception area.

    _____ 2. Go to the gym for an energizing yoga class twice a week after work.

    _____ 3. Keep up an ability to see the humor in life's events.

    _____ 4. Join your local chapter of the AAMA and participate in continuing education activities so you will have the CEUs you need to recertify.

    _____ 5. Keep a list of any special patient problems or needs by reviewing patient charts before formal office hours begin.

    _____ 6. Take a walk in a local park during a scheduled morning break.

    _____ 7. Learn how to practice self-motivation on tasks performed independently; feel free to contribute ideas and comments on group projects.

3. List and define the five considerations important in determining a goal.

    (1) _____

    _____

    (2) _____

    _____

(3) _____

_____

(4) _____

_____

(5) _____

_____

4. For each consideration important in determining a goal, list a personal goal of your own that meets its particular requirements. Choose different goals for each answer; do not use the same goal twice.

(1) _____

_____

(2) _____

_____

(3) _____

_____

(4) _____

_____

(5) _____

_____

5. Burnout is stress-related energy depletion that takes place in the working world. In the military world, burnout is called *battle fatigue*. Burnout occurs gradually over a period of continued stress.

Place a P next to those items that promote burnout and an R next to those that reduce the risk for burnout.

_____ 1. Keep work separate from your home life.

_____ 2. Have regular physical examinations.

_____ 3. Work harder than anyone else in the office.

_____ 4. Feel a greater need than others to do a job well for its own sake.

_____ 5. Prioritize tasks and perform the most difficult ones first.

_____ 6. Prefer to tackle projects yourself rather than consult a supervisor.

_____ 7. Never stop until you achieve your goals, regardless of the personal cost to yourself or loved ones.

_____ 8. Postpone vacation time.

_____ 9. Give up unrealistic goals and expectations.

_____ 10. Maintain a positive self-image and your self-esteem.

_____ 11. Develop interests outside your profession.

_____ 12. Procrastinate.

_____ 13. Wear loose-fitting, comfortable clothes and shoes.

_____ 14. Stretch or change positions. Walk around and deliver charts or laboratory specimens.

_____ 15. Know your limits and be aware of your body's needs.

6. The "wear and tear" our bodies experience as we continually adjust to a changing environment is called:

    a. adaptation

    b. stress

    c. prioritizing

    d. conditioning

7. The fight-or-flight response includes all but which one of the following reactions?

    a. respirations and heart rate increases

    b. digestion is activated

    c. hormones are released into the bloodstream

    d. blood supply is increased to the muscles

8. One of the characteristics associated with burnout is when the employee does not know what is expected and how to accomplish it. This is often called:

    a. role conflict

    b. role overload

    c. role ambiguity

    d. role reversal

9. When individuals with a high need to achieve do not reach their goals, they are apt to feel:

    a. angry and frustrated

    b. tired and lonely

    c. distrustful and leery

    d. motivated and enthusiastic

10. The best way to treat burnout is to:

    a. cover it up

    b. get a prescription to help you cope

    c. prevent it

    d. encourage it

CERTIFICATION REVIEW

These questions are designed to mimic the certification examinations. You can use these questions like a small "Certification Examination Study Guide," but this is not meant to take the place of the more extensive study guides. Use this portion to determine where to concentrate your efforts when studying for the certification examination.

1. The body's response to mental or physical change is called:
   a. stress
   b. adaptation
   c. denial
   d. burnout

2. Which of the following is not part of Hans Selye's general adaptation syndrome?
   a. exhaustion
   b. alarm
   c. fear
   d. fight or flight
   e. return to normal

3. The four parts of the process leading to burnout are the Honeymoon stage, the Reality stage, the Dissatisfaction stage, and the:
   a. Sad stage
   b. Angry stage
   c. Retaliation stage
   d. Giving Up stage

CASE STUDY

Angie Esposito is a physician at Inner City Health Care. It was her dream, even as a child, to become a physician and work in an environment where she could help people and benefit the community as well. Proud of her accomplishments, she is the first woman in her family to attend college, and she got herself through medical school with scholarships and student loans. Angie works hard, often pulling double shifts. Liz Corbin, CMA, has a similar dream and is working to save money to attend medical school to become a pediatrician. Dr. Esposito does her best to encourage Liz's ambitions and has taken Liz under her wing.

Late one night, Liz assists Dr. Esposito in treating three difficult emergency patients in a row. "That's it," Angie Esposito says. "We're taking a 15-minute break. Ask Dr. Woo if he can cover for a short time." When Liz catches up with Dr. Esposito in the employee lounge, she finds Angie in frustrated tears. "These double shifts," Angie says. "I'm so tired. And the patients just keep coming. I want to help them all," she sighs and her voice trails off, "I just can't help them all…"

Discuss the following:
1. Dr. Angie Esposito is experiencing burnout. What personality traits are promoting her burnout? Identify the stressors in Angie's life.
2. Liz Corbin, CMA, sees her mentor breaking down under stress. Should Liz reevaluate her own long-range goals?
3. Discuss the importance of keeping goals in perspective.
4. What is Liz's best therapeutic response to Dr. Esposito?

SELF-ASSESSMENT

Determining how well you now handle stress will help you to identify personal strengths and weaknesses and point you toward the skills you will need to develop to be successful on the job as a medical assistant. Complete the following stress self-test.

For each question, circle the response that best describes you.

1. I exercise:
   a. three times a week
   b. less than three times a week
   c. only if I am forced to

2. When something stressful happens in my life, I:
   a. eat too much
   b. make sure I eat regular meals
   c. stop eating for days

3. If I am struggling with a problem or project, I am most likely to:
   a. consult someone who may be able to help
   b. become determined to solve the problem or finish the project on my own
   c. abandon the project or just hope the problem goes away

4. When I encounter difficult personalities, I:
   a. leave the scene and avoid the person in the future
   b. lose my temper and get into arguments
   c. practice the art of the diplomatic response

5. When offered a new challenge or responsibility that requires obtaining new skills or training, I:
   a. get tension headaches
   b. respond with enthusiasm and an open mind
   c. express concern about taking on a new duty

6. In emergency situations, I:
   a. react calmly and efficiently
   b. feel paralyzed
   c. wait for someone else to take charge

7. I feel confident and competent in group situations:
   a. only when I know everyone present
   b. most of the time
   c. hardly ever; conversations with others make me uncomfortable

8. I think meditating or taking time to be quiet and calm during a busy day is:
   a. a terrific waste of time: I always have to be doing something
   b. good for other people: I've tried it more than once, but I can't seem to get into meditation
   c. a great way to relax and refocus my mind

9. The key to handling stressful situations lies in:
   a. staying out of stressful situations
   b. examining my view of the situation from a new direction
   c. insisting that everyone agree with my point of view

10. To accomplish my personal goals, I:
    a. am willing to get up an hour earlier each day
    b. will give up sleep altogether
    c. find myself losing sleep because I am worrying about how I am going to get everything done

11. I usually complete projects:
    a. on time
    b. at the last minute
    c. late—but only by a day

12. As I prepare for a day's activities, I:
    a. prioritize and use time management skills to budget time carefully
    b. do not prepare; I like to be spontaneous
    c. find myself overwhelmed and unable to complete anything

13. When I focus on setting a long-range goal, I:
    a. think through the short-range goals necessary to achieve it
    b. become impatient
    c. talk constantly about the goal without making plans to achieve it

14. I volunteer to take on:
    a. more tasks than any one person can easily accomplish—then amaze everyone by pulling them off
    b. only what I know I can reasonably accomplish
    c. only what is required to get the job done

15. After a stressful day, the best way to unwind is to:
    a. talk all night with family or friends about what happened
    b. rent a funny movie
    c. work late to prepare for tomorrow

16. People think of me as:
    a. a person who is unpredictable. No one knows what I will do next
    b. someone fixed in life roles
    c. someone who is confident about who I am, but who also is willing to grow and change as worthy opportunities arise

Scoring: In the "My Score" column, record the number of points earned for each of your answers. The higher your score, the less you are prone to stress. The highest possible score is 160 points. If your score is low, consider the areas you need to focus on to reduce stress in your life.

My Score | My Score

1. a. 10 points   b. 5 points   c. 0 point   _____
   Regular exercise reduces stress.

2. a. 0 point   b. 10 points   c. 0 point   _____
   Eating regular meals reduces stress.

3. a. 10 points   b. 5 points   c. 0 point   _____
   Problems rarely just go away; ask for help before struggling on your own.

4. a. 5 points   b. 0 point   c. 10 points   _____
   You won't always be able to avoid a difficult person, and argument leads to stress. Tact and grace are needed.

5. a. 0 point   b. 10 points   c. 5 points   _____
   Worrying to the point of causing physical symptoms is not productive. Close-mindedness could keep you from enjoying something new and cause stressful reactions.

6. a. 10 points   b. 0 point   c. 5 points   _____
   Feelings of helplessness increase stress.

7. a. 5 points   b. 10 points   c. 0 point   _____
   The ability to interact comfortably with others in group situations reduces stress.

8. a. 0 point   b. 5 points   c. 10 points   _____
   The more you can separate your sense of well-being from daily events by taking time to relax and refocus, the less stress you will experience.

9. a. 0 point   b. 10 points   c. 0 points   _____
   Stressful situations cannot always be avoided; keeping a flexible instead of a rigid viewpoint will reduce stress.

10. a. 10 points   b. 0 point   c. 0 point   _____
    Sleep is important in reducing stress. However, making time by getting up earlier is a good time-management technique.

11. a. 10 points   b. 5 points   c. 0 point   _____
    Lateness causes stress for everyone.

12. a. 10 points   b. 0 points   c. 0 point   _____
    Unexpected things can always happen, but prioritizing and budgeting time can help keep a handle on the day's events and reduce stress.

13. a. 10 points   b. 5 points   c. 0 point   _____
    Achieving long-range goals takes perseverance and determination. Being realistic about goals reduces stress.

14. a. 0 point   b. 10 points   c. 5 points   _____
    Taking on too much responsibility leads to stress.

15. a. 0 point   b. 10 points   c. 0 point   _____
    Humor is an effective stress reducer—so is separating work from your home life.

16. a. 0 point   b. 0 point   c. 10 points   _____
    Being grounded but open to new experiences reduces stress.

Total   _____

CHAPTER POST-TEST

This is similar to your Pre-Test. Perform this test without looking at the book. This is just to see how well you have understood and can recall the information presented in this chapter after you have studied it and completed the workbook exercises. You will not be graded on this portion (other than the grade you give yourself), but this is an excellent preparation for your instructor's test. You may use this Post-Test to determine what areas you need to study more. Justify any "false" answers.

1. Stress is never a good thing. (T or F)

2. Stress is something we can always prevent. (T or F)

3. Even if you have a lot of responsibility at work, you can still avoid burnout. (T or F)

4. Setting goals eliminates stress (T or F)

EVALUATION OF CHAPTER KNOWLEDGE

Evaluate your ability to identify your personal stressors and coping abilities.

Skills	Student Self-Evaluation		
	Good	Average	Poor
I can identify my personal short- and long-range goals.	———	———	———
I recognize my personal strengths and weaknesses in responding to stress.	———	———	———
I recognize inner- and outer-directed qualities of personal character.	———	———	———
I can describe physiologic effects of stress.	———	———	———
I understand behaviors that promote or reduce the risk for burnout.	———	———	———
I can differentiate between stress and stressors.	———	———	———
I can identify stressors common in the ambulatory care setting.	———	———	———

CHAPTER 6

The Therapeutic Approach to the Patient with a Life-Threatening Illness

CHAPTER PRE-TEST

Perform this test without looking at the book. This is just to see how well you have understood and can recall the information in this chapter after you have read it, but before you have completed the workbook exercises. You will not be graded on this portion (other than the grade you give yourself). Justify any "false" answers.

1. Patients from different cultures will view death and life-threatening illnesses in different ways. (T or F)

2. The strongest influences in managing life-threatening illnesses in the life of the patient comes from the medical team. (T or F)

3. Health care professionals are responsible for making sure that patients have all their legal documents in order when diagnosed with a life-threatening illness. (T or F)

4. Alternative methods of treatment should be discussed with the patient, as well as no treatment at all. (T or F)

5. When facing a life-threatening illness, setting goals is no longer important. (T or F)

INTRODUCTION

As a member of the health care team, the medical assistant will be involved in the care of patients with life-threatening illnesses. In addition to providing medical, surgical, and psychological care, the health care team relies on its skills of empathy and compassion in building a strong therapeutic approach to the treatment and care of patients with life-threatening illness. As a source of information for these patients and their families and significant others, medical assistants need to be sensitive, supportive, and respectful of people who have a life-threatening disease. It is important for medical assistants to remain impartial and professional, making patients as comfortable and confident as possible in the ambulatory care setting.

PERFORMANCE OBJECTIVES

After successful completion of this chapter you will be able to discuss the needs, both legal and emotional, of patients facing life-threatening illnesses. You will be familiar with the feelings the patients might be experiencing and be able to sympathize and empathize with them and their families. You will recognize the influences of various cultures regarding death and dying. You will have an understanding and an ability to assist patients who are experiencing life-threatening situations. Try not to look back at the textbook as you fill in the blanks in the following paragraph. If necessary, reread the textbook chapter. *The following statements are related to your learning objectives for this chapter. Fill in the blanks with the appropriate term(s):*

Everything learned in the previous chapter about therapeutic communication is heightened and considerably more difficult when the patient has a (1) _____ _____ _____.

It is essential for the medical assistant to recognize that the (2) _____ of the patients will change when handling a life-threatening illness. No two individuals will respond to a life-threatening illness in the same way. Some patients will respond with (3) _____. Some patients will prepare for death by altering their lives drastically. Some patients will quietly continue their lives with little obvious (4) _____. Although the health care professionals are not (5) _____ for providing legal advice and documents for the patient, it is in the best interest of the patient and the health care team to raise topics for discussion during the course of the patient's life-threatening illness.

VOCABULARY BUILDER

Find the word below that is misspelled; circle it, and then correctly spell it in the space provided. Then insert the correct vocabulary terms from the list that best fit the descriptions below.

durible power of attorney for health care

living will

physician's directive

psychomotor retardation

_____

1. _____ allows the surrogate to make decisions related to health care when the patient is no longer able to do so.

2. _____ and _____ allow the patients to make decisions (before becoming incapacitated) of whether life-prolonging medical or surgical procedures are to continue or be withheld.

3. _____ is the slowing of mental responses, decreased alertness, and apathy.

Crossword Puzzle

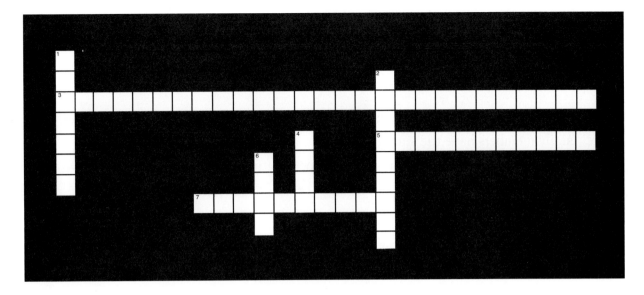

Across

3. This 1990 Act gave all patients in institutions that were Medicare or Medicaid funded certain rights
5. Aiding health, healthful
7. This emotion is common in patients dealing with life-threatening illnesses

Down

1. Recognition of another person's feelings by entering into those feelings
2. This type of support is vital when dealing with a life-threatening illness
4. Late stages of HIV infection
6. End-stage renal disease

LEARNING REVIEW

1. List five issues that are appropriate to discuss with a patient facing a life-threatening illness.

   (a) _____

   (b) _____

   (c) _____

   (d) _____

   (e) _____

2. Discuss the pros and cons of using the words terminal illness or life-threatening illness. Which term seems more comfortable to you? Defend your rationale.

3. The federal government passed the Patient Self-Determination Act in _____, giving all patients receiving care in institutions that receive payments from Medicare and Medicaid written information about their right to accept or refuse medical or surgical treatment.

   a. 1962

   b. 1990

   c. 1998

   d. 1973

4. What patients fear, more than anything else, when facing a life-threatening illness is:
   a. pain and loss of independence
   b. dementia
   c. financial issues
   d. becoming addicted to some medications

5. In caring for individuals with life-threatening illnesses, it can be helpful to remember:
   a. family members have the strongest influences on patients
   b. pain must be considered within a cultural perspective
   c. choices and decisions regarding treatment belong to the patient
   d. all of the above

6. One of the most common problems that a patient with life-threatening illness may exhibit is:
   a. displacement
   b. denial
   c. depression
   d. assimilation

7. Referrals to community-based agencies or service groups may include:
   a. health departments
   b. social workers
   c. hospice
   d. all of the above

CERTIFICATION REVIEW

These questions are designed to mimic the certification examinations. You can use these questions like a small "Certification Examination Study Guide," but this is not meant to take the place of the more extensive study guides. Use this portion to determine where to concentrate your efforts when studying for the certification examination.

1. Your patient's culture influences:
   a. his or her views on illness
   b. his or her views about treatment
   c. his or her views about death
   d. all of the above

2. When a person is faced with a life-threatening illness, he or she will go through certain stages of grieving. (T or F)

3. Your patient has just been diagnosed with a life-threatening illness. She tells you that she would much rather die quickly than to suffer through this disease. She asks you not to say anything about her comment to the doctor. What is your best response?

  a. You have had quite a shock. Dr. King would like to talk to you about those feelings. I'll go get him for you.

  b. You, above anyone else, know what is best for your life.

  c. I know what you mean, I would feel the same way

  d. Don't worry about that right now. Dr. King will give you medication to help with the pain.

CASE STUDIES

In working with patients with life-threatening illnesses, medical assistants hone their personal coping skills, capitalizing on strengths, maintaining hope, and showing continued human care and concern. For each case scenario presented, answer the following questions:

  1. What is the best therapeutic response of the medical assistant?
  2. On what criteria do you base this response as the best therapeutic approach?

Case 1

Jaime Carrera, a Hispanic man in his late 20s, is brought to Inner City Health Care, an urgent care center, by coworkers when he injures his head in an accident at a construction site where he is working. His head is bleeding profusely. As Jaime's coworkers watch the health care team implement Standard Precautions for infection control, one of them, his own shirt and hands covered with Jaime's blood, pulls the medical assistant aside and whispers frantically, "What are you doing? Does he have AIDS?"

Case 2

John Dukane, a longtime and much loved patient of the clinic, has end-stage renal disease. A kidney transplant is not appropriate, and his age of 83 years has led John to determine that he will not choose renal dialysis as a treatment. That decision has been made clear in his physician's directive and durable power of attorney for health care. He is healthy otherwise, and his family members think he should try the dialysis, which could extend his life a few weeks or months. Discuss the arguments on both sides of the decision.

SELF-ASSESSMENT

  1. If you were faced with a life-threatening illness, would you choose to sustain your life regardless of the probable outcome? How far would you go with treatments? What four factors would enter into your decision? Have you discussed these issues with your family and physician?

CHAPTER POST-TEST

This is similar to the Pre-Test. Perform this test without looking at the book. This is just to see how well you have understood and can recall the information presented in this chapter after you have studied it and completed the workbook exercises. You will not be graded on this portion (other than the grade you give yourself), but this is an excellent preparation for your instructor's test. You may use this Post-Test to determine what areas you need to study more. Justify any "false" answers.

1. Patients view death and life-threatening illnesses in different ways depending on their culture. (T or F)

2. The strongest influences in managing life-threatening illnesses in the life of the patient comes from his or her family members. (T or F)

3. Health care professionals are not responsible for making sure that patients have all their legal documents in order when diagnosed with a life-threatening illness. (T or F)

4. Alternative methods of treatment, as well as the option of no treatment at all, should be discussed with the patient. (T or F)

5. When facing a life-threatening illness, setting goals is still important. (T or F)

CERTIFICATION CRITERIA CHECKLIST

As you go through your education and training, keep in mind the national certification examination that you will take when you graduate. Each chapter of the textbook and workbook covers a different section of the examination criteria. To keep track of your preparation for the certification examination, turn to the back of this workbook and highlight the following CMA, RMA, or CMAS certification examination criteria (if you have already highlighted them from a previous chapter, put a check mark by the criteria):

CMA
C. Psychology
    1. Basic principles
    3. Hereditary, cultural and environmental influences on behavior
E. Communication
    1. Adapting communication to an individual's ability to understand
    4. Professional communication and behavior
    5. Evaluating and understanding communication
M. Resource Information and Community Services
    4. Patient advocate

RMA
I. General Medical Assisting Knowledge
    E. Human Relations
        1. Patient relations
        2. Interpersonal relations
    F. Patient Resource Materials

CMAS
1. Medical Assisting Foundation
    • Professionalism

EVALUATION OF CHAPTER KNOWLEDGE

Evaluate your own strengths and weaknesses in administering a therapeutic approach to the patient with a life-threatening illness.

Skills	Student Self-Evaluation		
	Good	Average	Poor
I can recognize psychological problems that accompany life-threatening illnesses.	——	——	——
I can identify my personal fears or concerns about assisting in the care and treatment of patients with life-threatening illnesses.	——	——	——
I have the ability to treat patients and families with empathy, impartiality, and respect.	——	——	——
I recognize the demands of providing therapeutic care for patients with life-threatening illnesses in the ambulatory care setting.	——	——	——
I have the skills to avoid emotional burnout when caring for patients with life-threatening illnesses.	——	——	——
I understand the use of Standard Precautions for infection control in protecting myself.	——	——	——

CHAPTER 7

Legal Considerations

CHAPTER PRE-TEST

Perform this test without looking at the book. This is just to see how well you have understood and can recall the information in this chapter after you have read it, but before you have completed the workbook exercises. You will not be graded on this portion (other than the grade you give yourself). Justify any "false" answers.

1. You may discuss a person's confidential medical information as long as you do not say the patient's name. (T or F)

2. Your physician does not have a contract with the patient until he or she treats the patient. (T or F)

3. A physician practicing medicine without a license would come under (*circle one*): criminal law or civil law?

4. A physician may stop treating a patient immediately if the patient refuses to pay his or her bill. (T or F)

5. Medical assistants do not have to worry about a "standard of care" because their physician–employers are ultimately responsible for everything the medical assistant does under their direction. (T or F)

INTRODUCTION

Medical assistants and other health care professionals are employed in the medical profession, where laws regulate medical and business practices at both the state and the federal levels. Regulatory agencies act to investigate the quality of health care and control health care costs while providing equitable access to care. Medical assistants need to be aware of the laws and regulations that govern the practices and procedures followed by health care professionals in the ambulatory care setting. In a society that strongly advocates the individual's right to seek redress in a court of law, the potential for litigation in medical settings must be considered. As responsible health care professionals, medical assistants need to understand the regulations and laws that affect their daily experiences on the job and to behave appropriately within the scope of their training and knowledge.

PERFORMANCE OBJECTIVES

After successful completion of this chapter you will be able to discuss the four sources of law, compare civil law with criminal law, and identify the three major areas of civil law that affect the medical profession. You will be able to recall at least seven of the nine administrative laws important to the medical profession. You will be able to define administering, prescribing, and dispensing medications and cite how these actions are applied to controlled substances. You will know three main goals of the Health Insurance Portability and Accountability Act (HIPAA), the differences between implied and expressed contracts; the three main reasons for the physician–patient contract to be terminated and how to go about instituting a termination. You will be able to discuss torts, the four Ds of negligence, and what constitutes battery in the ambulatory care setting; describe two forms of defamation of character; and cite at least 10 practices to help in risk management. You will be able to discuss informed consent, the types of minors, the necessary steps in a civil litigation, and how a medical assistant might be involved. You will understand subpoenas and be able to recall special issues of confidentiality, statute of limitations, public duties, and AIDS. *The following statements are related to your learning objectives for this chapter. Fill in the blanks in the following paragraphs with the appropriate term(s).*

Law may come from five different sources: (1) _____, (2) _____, (3) _____, (4) _____, and (5) _____. The main difference between civil and criminal law is that civil law addresses crimes (6) _____, and criminal law addresses crimes (7) _____. The three major areas of civil law that affect the medical profession are (8) _____, (9) _____ _____, and (10) _____. Three main goals of HIPAA are (11) _____, (12) _____, and (13) _____. Medical assistants are considered (14) _____ of the physicians they serve and as such should be cautious in their actions and (15) _____. A physician is obligated to continue care on a patient unless one of three things happens: The (16) _____ may discharge the physician, the (17) _____ formally withdraws, or the (18) _____ no longer (19) _____ _____. A (20) _____ law is a wrongful act, other than a breach of contract, resulting in injury to one person by another. The four Ds of negligence are: (21) _____, (22) _____, (23) _____, and (24) _____. The touching of another person without their consent is considered (25) _____. Defamation of character consists of the injury of another person's (26) _____, (27) _____, or (28) _____, either through (29) _____ or (30) _____ words. Consent may be either (31) _____ or implied. Implied consent may occur when the patient is in a life-threatening situation or when the patient is (32) _____ or unable to respond. Implied consent may also occur in more

(33) _____ ways. Persons who are under the age of 18 years, but are free from parental care are called (34) _____ _____. You may be protected from being sued if you give first aid at the scene of an accident provided you stay within your (35) _____.

VOCABULARY BUILDER

Find the words below that are misspelled; circle them, and then correctly spell them in the spaces provided. Then insert the correct vocabulary terms from the list that best fit the descriptions below.

A. agents
B. civil law
C. malfeasance
D. defendents
E. doctrins
F. durable power of attorney for health care
G. emanciated minor
H. expert witness

I. expressed contract
J. implied consent
K. constitutional law
L. incompetant
M. lible
N. litigation
O. malpractice
P. administrative law
Q. miner

R. negligance
S. noncompliant
T. plaintiffs
U. risk management
V. slander
W. statutes
X. supoena
Y. tort

_____   _____   _____

_____   _____   _____

_____   _____

1.____ Establishes agencies given power to enact regulations having the force of law

2.____ Designation of health care surrogate

3.____ Law that includes 27 amendments, 10 of which are the Bill of Rights

4.____ A 17-year-old person serving in the U.S. armed forces

5.____ Medical practice acts, or laws, that regulate the practice of medicine, such as licensure and standards of care

6.____ A patient who refuses needed care, such as a cancer patient who will not complete a series of chemotherapy treatments

7.____ A physician or health care professional who testifies in court to establish a reasonable and expected standard of care with respect to a specific medical situation so that jurors can understand the nature of medical information

8.____ The failure to exercise the standard of care that a reasonable person would exercise in similar circumstances

9.____ A patient sues a laboratory for money damages for delivering an incorrect analysis of a specimen that results in misdiagnosis by a physician

10.____ In a state where medical assistants must be licensed to perform venipuncture, charges are brought against a person who is performing this invasive procedure without the proper licensure

11.____ Persons who bring charges in a civil case

12.____ Medical assistants are _____ of their physician–employers

13.____ A written lease for office space

14._____ A patient tilts her head back and opens her eyes wide for instillation of medicated eye-drops from a medical assistant without any verbal instructions to do so

15._____ Professional negligence

16._____ *Respondeat superior* and *res ipsa loquitur*

17._____ Although the patient, a competent adult, forcibly draws back, the medical assistant proceeds to administer an injection, breaking off the needle in the skin

18._____ Court order

19._____ Persons against whom charges are brought

20._____ A medical assistant writes in the patient's record, "Jim Marshall is a ruthless, rude man who is very full of himself. Be careful around him."

21._____ A patient says loudly in the reception area of Inner City Health Care, filled to capacity with waiting patients, "Dr. Reynolds should retire. I know he's not up on the latest medical techniques."

22._____ Lawsuit

23._____ A 17-year-old student who lives with his or her parents

24._____ A person found by the court to be insane, inadequate, or not an adult

25._____ Actions that make the medical assistant and the physician–employer less vulnerable to litigations

Crossword Puzzle

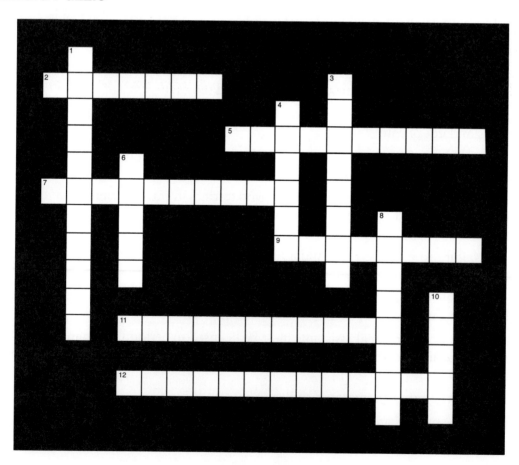

Clues

Across

2. The type of consent that is given when a patient is unconscious
5. When a doctor should have treated a patient, but did not, it can sometimes be called this
7. Another word for lawsuit
9. Another word for laws
11. A type of lawsuit in which the doctor is accused of harming a patient
12. When a patient does not follow the doctor's orders, such as not taking medication that is prescribed

Down

1. Minors (under 18 years old) who are no longer under parental authority
3. Law that governs criminal acts
4. Medical assistants are ___ of our physician–employers
6. Law that governs issues between persons
8. This document is a legal force that you must comply with
10. When someone harms another person's reputation by saying something untrue

LEARNING REVIEW

1. Civil law is a branch of the law in which restitution is awarded to individuals, usually in monetary form, when a civil wrong has been committed. Crimes against the safety and welfare of society as a whole, however, are addressed by criminal law, in which the punishment is usually incarceration and/or a fine.

   Identify whether the following actions fall under the domain of civil law (CV) or criminal law (CM).

   _____ A. A physician is siphoning off narcotics from an urgent care center's locked drug cabinet and continuing to treat patients while under the influence of the drugs.

   _____ B. A woman, in the advanced stages of breast cancer, sues her insurer when it refuses to provide benefits for a bone marrow transplant.

   _____ C. An office manager steals, or embezzles, funds from the medical practice.

2. Contracts are expressed or implied. Expressed contracts are written or verbal agreements that specify the exact duties of each party. Implied contracts depend on the power of action and circumstance; the actions performed would have been intended had an expressed contract existed.

   Identify each of the following as an expressed (E), implied (I), or invalid (X) contract.

   _____ A. professional negligence contract

   _____ B. living will

   _____ C. rescue breathing

   _____ D. patient appointment scheduled over the telephone

   _____ E. a purchase order for office supplies

   _____ F. completing a consent form for major abdominal surgery

   _____ G. a physician's directive signed by a patient with progressive Alzheimer's disease

   _____ H. a medical decision made by a health care surrogate for a patient suffering a debilitating cerebral vascular accident (CVA)

   _____ I. setting the fractured arm of a 6-year-old child rushed to the emergency department after a playground fall, and the parent has not consented

   _____ J. confirming verbal acceptance of a job offer as a clinical medical assistant by a handshake with the office manager of the medical practice

3. List and define the four Ds of negligence.

   (1) _____

   _____

   (2) _____

   _____

   (3) _____

   _____

   (4) _____

   _____

4. List at least 11 strategies for risk management in an ambulatory care setting that will lessen the potential for litigation.

   (1) _____

   _____

   (2) _____

   _____

   (3) _____

   _____

   (4) _____

   _____

   (5) _____

   _____

   (6) _____

   _____

   (7) _____

   _____

   (8) _____

   _____

   (9) _____

   _____

   (10) _____

   _____

   (11) _____

   _____

5. Before any invasive or surgical procedure is performed, patients are asked to sign consent forms, which become a permanent part of the medical record. What four things must the patient know to give informed consent?

    (1) _____

    (2) _____

    (3) _____

    (4) _____

6. The unauthorized touching of one person by another is:

    a. invasion of privacy

    b. defamation

    c. libel

    d. battery

7. The federal government established laws in 1968 to allow people to make a gift of all or part of their body. It is known as:

    a. Occupational Safety and Health Act (OSHA)

    b. Uniform Anatomical Gift Act

    c. Family Gift Act

    d. Death Act of 1968

    e. Body Right Act of 1968

8. Protection of health care professionals who may provide medical care in an emergency without fear of being sued is called the:

    a. Good Samaritan laws

    b. physician's directives

    c. durable power of attorney for health care

    d. litigation

9. The law mandates that certain diseases and injuries are reported to the proper authorities; these include:

    a. rape

    b. gunshot and knife wounds

    c. child abuse

    d. elder abuse

    e. all of the above

    f. c and d only

10. An order for a physician to appear in court with a medicine record is:

    a. *res ipsa loquitur*

    b. *subpoena duces tecum*

    c. *respondeat superior*

    d. an interrogatory

CERTIFICATION REVIEW

These questions are designed to mimic the certification examinations. You can use these questions like a small "Certification Examination Study Guide," but this is not meant to take the place of the more extensive study guides. Use this portion to determine which areas to concentrate your efforts when studying for the certification examination.

1. The Patient's Self-Determination Act, which includes advanced directives, is to ensure that patients are able to:
    a. choose their own physician
    b. control their own health care decisions
    c. have guaranteed confidentiality
    d. have health care benefits

2. Which of the following covers the relationship between physicians and their patients?
    a. informed consent
    b. locum tenens
    c. medical ethics
    d. contract law

3. *Res ipsa loquitur* means:
    a. the thing speaks for itself
    b. the physician is ultimately responsible
    c. the record must be opened in court
    d. patients have a right to their records

4. The 4 Ds of negligence are:
    a. duty, dereliction, danger, damage
    b. danger, duty, direct cause, disaster
    c. duty, dereliction, direct cause, damage
    d. disaster, damage, direct cause, disaster

5. A 17-year-old individual who is in the navy is considered to be:
    a. *respondeat superior*
    b. an emancipated minor
    c. privileged
    d. a naval dependent

CASE STUDIES

For each of the following cases, what errors are made that could leave the medical assistants and physician-employers vulnerable to litigation? How might the errors leave the health care professionals open to potential lawsuits? How could the errors have been avoided through effective risk management techniques?

Case 1

On a busy afternoon at Inner City Health Care, the reception area is filled with walk-in patients and the staff struggles to keep up with the patient load. Administrative medical assistant Liz Corbin, CMA, gives the patient file for Edith Leonard to clinical medical assistant Bruce Goldman, CMA. "Dr. Reynolds wants a CBC done stat on the older adult woman in exam room 1," she tells Bruce, handing him the file.

Bruce proceeds to examination room 1; without identifying the patient, he performs a venipuncture on Cele Little, who has come to the clinic for a hearing problem. Cele asks Bruce why the procedure needs to be performed and doesn't want to have it. Bruce insists that the physician has ordered the procedure and performs the venipuncture anyway. The procedure frightens Cele, and she begins to fear her hearing loss is indicative of a more serious illness.

Case 2

Dr. Elizabeth King has just completed a routine physical examination of Abigail Johnson. Elizabeth asks Anna Preciado, RMA, to administer a flu shot to Abigail before she leaves the office. Abigail, an older African-American woman, is accompanied by her daughter. When Anna attempts to administer the flu vaccine, Abigail says, "Is that a flu shot? They make me sick; I don't want it."

Abigail's daughter says, "Yes, she does want it. Go ahead and give it to her."

Abigail begins to laugh. "Okay," Anna says, "may I give you the vaccination?"

Abigail says nothing, but she rolls up her sleeve. As Anne administers the parenteral injection, the older woman looks up at her seriously and says, "I didn't want any flu shot. My daughter makes me get it every year." However, Abigail does not withdraw physically.

Case 3

Dr. Elizabeth King is going over the daily list of scheduled patients with Ellen Armstrong, CMA. They are standing at the front desk close to the reception area; several patients are waiting for the first appointments of the day. Elizabeth's eye moves down the list and stops over the name Mary O'Keefe. "Mary O'Keefe," she mutters, "she's so neurotic and pestering. It's a small wonder her husband hasn't left her yet; just wait till they have that third child. . . . I don't think I have the patience for Mary today."

Case 4

Lydia Renzi, a deaf woman with some residual hearing, comes to Inner City Health Care with a recurrent vaginal discharge. Lydia is diagnosed by Dr. Angie Esposito with candidiasis, a yeast infection caused by the fungus *Candida albicans*; Angie prescribes a vaginal suppository and asks Wanda Slawson, CMA, to give Lydia instructions for using the prescription. Lydia wears a hearing aid and has chosen not to be accompanied to the clinic by a sign language interpreter. Lydia has trouble understanding Wanda, who is soft spoken; Wanda is also standing against a brightly lit window, and Lydia has trouble seeing her face. Lydia writes on a pad she has brought with her, "Is this a sexually transmitted illness?"

In frustration, Wanda begins shouting, "You just have a yeast infection; it's not like you have herpes or anything." At that moment, Bruce Goldman, CMA, is escorting a male patient past the open door of the examination room. Both men turn their heads away, though it is clear they have overheard.

Case 5

Construction workers Jaime Carrera and Ralph Samson are required to take a preemployment drug-screening test before they can be hired to work on a new site to which they have applied. Jaime and Ralph come to Inner City Health Care, where urine specimens are collected for examination. The test comes back positive for Jaime, and his potential employer does not give him the job. Ralph tests negative. Two weeks later, Ralph returns to Inner City Health Care for a routine physical examination.

"Whatever happened to Jaime Carrera?" Ralph asks Bruce Goldman, CMA. "I haven't seen him around the site."

"Oh," Bruce replies, "he tested positive for chemical substance abuse, and now he's in a rehab program Dr. Whitney suggested."

SELF ASSESSMENT

1. Have you ever been in a situation in which you were asked to disclose information about another person that might have been considered confidential? Or have you ever been told confidential information? If this has happened (or if it happens in the future), what should you have done or said? What will you do/say in the future?

CHAPTER POST-TEST

This is similar to your Pre-Test. Perform this test without looking at the book. This is just to see how well you have understood and can recall the information presented in this chapter after you have studied it and completed the workbook exercises. You will not be graded on this portion (other than the grade you give yourself), but this is an excellent preparation for your instructor's test. You may use this Post-Test to determine where you need to study more. Justify any "false" answers.

1. As long as you do not say the patient's name you may discuss the patient's illnesses and treatments with anyone. (T or F)

2. The patient–physician contract begins when the patient makes the appointment. (T or F)

3. A physician practicing medicine without a license is breaking a *(circle one)*: criminal law or civil law.

4. If patients refuse to pay their bills, a physician may stop treating them immediately. (T or F)

5. Because our physician–employers are ultimately responsible for everything the medical assistant does under their direction, medical assistants do not have to worry about a "standard of care." (T or F)

CERTIFICATION CRITERIA CHECKLIST

As you go through your education and training, keep in mind the national certification examination that you will take when you graduate. Each chapter of the textbook and workbook covers a different section of the examination criteria. To keep track of your preparation for the certification examination, turn to the back of this workbook and highlight the following CMA, RMA, or CMAS certification examination criteria (if you have already highlighted them from a previous chapter, put a check mark by the criteria):

CMA

D.   Professionalism
      1.   Displaying professional attitude
      3.   Performing within ethical boundaries
      4.   Maintaining confidentiality
F.   Medicolegal Guidelines & Requirements
      1.   Licenses and accreditation
      2.   Legislation
      5.   Physician–patient relationship
M.   Resource Information and Community Services
      4.   Patient advocate

RMA

I.   General Medical Assisting Knowledge
      C.   Medical Law
            2. Licensure, certification, and registration
      E.   Medical Ethics
            1. Principles of medical ethics and ethical conduct

CMAS

1.   Medical Assisting Foundation
      •   Professionalism
      •   Legal and ethical considerations
4.   Medical Records Management
      •   Confidentiality
8.   Medical Office Management
      •   Risk management and quality assurance

EVALUATION OF CHAPTER KNOWLEDGE

Skills	Student Self-Evaluation		
	Good	Average	Poor
I can apply legal concepts to the ambulatory care setting.	_____	_____	_____
I understand the concept of standard of care.	_____	_____	_____
I can identify expressed and implied contracts.	_____	_____	_____
I understand informed consent.	_____	_____	_____
I recognize the need to practice effective risk management techniques.	_____	_____	_____
I understand the doctrine of *respondeat superior.*	_____	_____	_____
I can identify common torts in the ambulatory care setting.	_____	_____	_____
I can define malpractice and its components (4 Ds).	_____	_____	_____
I have a good working knowledge of Good Samaritan laws, the physician's directive, and the Americans with Disabilities Act.	_____	_____	_____
I understand accurate documentation requirements and reporting abuse.	_____	_____	_____

CHAPTER 8

Ethical Considerations

CHAPTER PRE-TEST

Perform this test without looking at the book. This is just to see how well you have understood and can recall the information in this chapter after you have read it, but before you have completed the workbook exercises. You will not be graded on this portion (other than the grade you give yourself). Justify any "false" answers.

1. Ethics has to do with what is right and wrong. (T or F)

2. Bioethics has to do with ethical issues dealing with human life. (T or F)

3. When abuse is suspected, the physician and medical assistant have ethical responsibilities to report it. (T or F)

4. When a patient has HIV, the physician may refuse to treat the patient. (T or F)

5. A physician and medical assistant can refuse to perform abortions. (T or F)

INTRODUCTION

Laws and regulations that govern the practice of medicine ensure that basic requirements and guidelines for protecting both patients and health care providers are observed. Medical assistants and all health care professionals are charged with the ethical responsibility to follow the law and to perform their duties within the scope of their training and practice. Laws and regulations find their origins in a system of ethics, or what is considered to be right and wrong behavior. As medical technology continues to advance, ethical dilemmas are created that challenge traditional codes of behavior. Medical ethics often confront ethical issues of great social controversy, such as in the field of bioethics. Medical assistants need to examine carefully their own deeply held values and beliefs, opinions, and their system of personal ethics, to build a strong foundation with which to face the ethical dilemmas encountered in the ambulatory care setting. We must strive to remain impartial and nonjudgmental in providing care.

PERFORMANCE OBJECTIVES

After successful completion of this chapter you will be able to discuss the reasons for a medical Code of Ethics, the eight characteristics of principle-centered leadership, the five Ps of ethical power, and the ethical guidelines for doctors, and you will be able to cite a few examples. You will be able to relate the five principles of the AAMA code to patient care and restate the dilemmas encountered in certain current bioethical issues. *The following statements are related to your learning objectives for this chapter. Fill in the blanks in the following paragraphs with the appropriate term(s).*

Another word for ethics might be (1) _____. Ethics are often identified in a set of principles and guidelines called (2) _____. The physician's code of ethics is called (3) _____. There are more than (4) _____ differ-ent codes of ethics; seven of them are worldwide. (5) _____ refers to those ethics that have to do with life issues such as abortion, fetal tissue research, right to die, among others.

VOCABULARY BUILDER

Find the words below that are misspelled; circle them, and then correctly spell them in the spaces provided. Then insert correct vocabulary terms from the list that best fit into the descriptive sentence below.

bioethics	genetic enginering	macroallocation
criopreservation	microallocation	serrogate
ethics		

_____   _____   _____

1. _____ Someone who substitutes for another

2. _____ Branch of ethics resulting from sophisticated medical research

3. _____ Medical decisions made by Congress

4. _____ Defined as a code of what is right or wrong

5. _____ Medical decisions made by individuals and physicians

6. _____ Biotechnology used to diagnose diseases, produce medicines, and so forth

7. _____ The use of freezing to preserve tissue for later use

Word Game

Find the words in the grid below. They may go in any direction. When you are finished, the first few unused letters in the grid will spell out a hidden message.

```
S  T  R  R  E  S  O  U  R  C  E  S  I  S  V  E  T
O  Y  M  D  C  E  O  W  H  A  T  I  C  S  M  M  E
O  G  I  R  O  S  R  E  W  O  P  I  A  A  L  L  N
L  O  C  Y  D  U  A  L  W  S  T  N  C  D  G  E  G
A  L  R  T  E  B  A  R  E  E  C  R  H  N  I  C  I
C  O  O  S  S  A  O  L  N  A  O  I  I  A  L  L  N
I  N  A  P  N  N  Y  E  L  A  D  S  H  R  I  M  E
H  H  L  R  G  O  G  G  L  O  I  E  S  T  O  H  E
T  C  L  O  T  L  I  L  G  T  C  A  R  R  E  Y  R
E  E  O  T  N  N  O  S  R  R  M  A  A  S  G  Q  I
O  T  C  E  K  C  T  E  I  M  I  L  T  P  H  W  N
I  O  A  C  A  L  V  P  E  C  L  G  L  I  Y  I  G
B  I  T  T  V  D  P  L  R  Y  E  N  H  P  O  R  P
T  B  I  I  A  Z  I  Y  M  V  V  D  G  T  N  N  W
M  O  O  N  N  D  L  Y  R  E  S  E  A  R  C  H  R
N  X  N  G  E  T  A  G  O  R  R  U  S  N  K  D  D
P  C  O  N  F  I  D  E  N  T  I  A  L  I  T  Y  G
```

abuse	dilemmas	power
advertising	engineering	protecting
allocation	ethics	research
bioethical	genetics	resources
biotechnology	leadership	right
codes	macroallocation	surrogate
confidentiality	microallocation	wrong
decisions	morally	

LEARNING REVIEW

1. The AAMA Code of Ethics presents five basic principles that medical assistants must pledge to honor as members of the medical assisting profession.

   For each situation presented, identify the AAMA ethical principle that applies.

   A. Render service with full respect for the dignity of humanity.

   B. Respect confidential information.

   C. Uphold the honor and integrity of the profession.

D. Pursue continuing education activities and improve knowledge and skills.

E. Participate in community service and education.

_____ 1. Marilyn Johnson, CMA, in conversation with co-office manager Shirley Brooks, CMA, refuses to speculate about whether a diagnosis of AIDS will be confirmed for patient Maria Jover.

_____ 2. Administrative medical assistant Karen Ritter joins a study group to prepare for the CMA certification examination as a method of securing her recertification of credentials, which is required every 5 years.

_____ 3. Clinical medical assistant Anna Preciado agrees to speak to a group of high school students who are interested in pursuing a career in the medical assisting profession.

_____ 4. Liz Corbin, CMA, politely reminds older adult patient Edith Leonard that she is a medical assistant, not a nurse, but assures Edith that she is qualified to perform the instillation of medicated eyedrops ordered by Dr. Susan Rice.

_____ 5. When patient Dottie Tate makes an appointment at Inner City Health Care for follow-up treatment of chronic back pain and a recent history of frequent falls, Bruce Goldman, CMA, prearranges for a wheelchair to accommodate Dottie's office visit.

_____ 6. Karen Ritter, CMA, volunteers at the local community office of Planned Parenthood on weekends.

_____ 7. Jane O'Hara, CMA, gently and kindly guides patient Wayne Elder, whose mild retardation often causes him to become confused in unfamiliar settings, back to the proper examination room when she finds him wandering down the hallway in search of Dr. Ray Reynolds.

_____ 8. When filing a group of recent laboratory reports into the correct patient files, Ellen Armstrong, CMA, takes care to complete the task quickly and efficiently. She performs the task at a private office station away from the general reception area and does not leave the charts open or unattended as she works.

_____ 9. Audrey Jones, CMA, approaches office manager Shirley Brooks, CMA, about opportunities for obtaining advanced training to become qualified to perform a wider array of clinical procedures in the ambulatory care setting.

_____ 10. Clinical medical assistant Wanda Slawson, who assisted Dr. Mark Woo in the treatment of patient Rhoda Au, diagnosed with lupus erythematosus, believes the patient is foolhardy when she rejects Mark's treatment plan of Western drug therapy in favor of an approach that integrates Chinese medicine. However, she respects the patient's heritage and right to choose her own health care.

2. According to the *Current Opinions of the Council on Ethical and Judicial Affairs of the AMA*, advertising by physicians is considered ethical if the ad follows certain requirements. Which of the following are appropriate types of physician advertisements? *Circle each correct response.*

A. Testimonials from patients cured of serious illnesses or whose conditions were reversed or controlled under the care and treatment of the physician.

B. Physicians' credentials, together with physicians' hospital or community affiliations.

   C. A description of the practice, facility hours of operation, and the types of services available to health care consumers.

   D. Photographs of health care professionals performing their duties at a medical facility. For example, a physical therapist applying ultrasound, a deep-tissue modality, to a patient experiencing chronic lower back pain.

   E. Guarantees of cure promised within a specific time frame.

   F. Word-of-mouth advertisement from patients.

3. Patient medical records are confidential legal documents. Name three instances, however, in which health professionals are allowed or required to reveal confidential patient information by law.

   (1) _____

   (2) _____

   (3) _____

4. Which state recently passed a physician-assisted suicide law?

   a. Florida

   b. California

   c. Oregon

   d. Texas

5. Revealing information about patients without consent unless otherwise required to do so by law is:

   a. a breach of confidentiality

   b. bioethics

   c. a conflict of interest

   d. genetic manipulation

6. Allocation of scarce resources may refer to:

   a. rationing of health care

   b. denied services

   c. advertising by health care professionals

   d. a and b only

7. *Roe v. Wade* refers to guidelines for:

   a. artificial insemination

   b. surrogacy

   c. abortion

   d. fetal tissue transplant

8. Codes of ethics:

   a. remain constant over time

   b. constantly change and evolve

   c. enhance professionalism

   d. are challenged and examined

   e. all but a

   f. none of the above

CERTIFICATION REVIEW

These questions are designed to mimic the certification examinations. You can use these questions like a small "Certification Examination Study Guide," but this is not meant to take the place of the more extensive study guides. Use this portion to determine in what areas to concentrate your efforts when studying for the certification examination.

1. The AAMA Code of Ethics includes all but which one of the following?

   a. We should render service with respect for the dignity of our patients.

   b. We should be paid an equitable salary/wage.

   c. We should respect confidential information.

   d. We should accept the disciplines of the profession.

   e. We should seek to improve our knowledge and skills.

2. Physicians may choose who to treat but may not refuse treatment based on certain criteria. Which of the following is untrue?

   a. Physicians may not refuse to treat patients based on race, color, religion, or national origin.

   b. It is unethical for a physician to refuse to treat a patient who is HIV-positive.

   c. Physicians must inform a patient's family of a patient's death and not delegate that responsibility to others.

   d. Physicians who know they are HIV-positive should tell their patients.

   e. Physicians should report unethical behaviors committed by other physicians.

CASE STUDY

Lourdes Austen arrives at the offices of Drs. Winston Lewis and Elizabeth King for her annual physical examination. It has been one year since Lourdes had surgery to remove a tumor in her breast by lumpectomy with axillary lymph node dissection, followed by a course of radiation. Lourdes's one-year mammogram and follow-up examinations with her surgeon and radiologist find no evidence of a recurrence of the cancer. Lourdes is a single woman in her late 30s. As Elizabeth begins the routine physical examination, assisted by Anna Preciado, RMA, Lourdes begins to cry. "I'm so happy to be alive," Lourdes says. "And so afraid of the cancer coming back. But I want to celebrate life. I've talked to my boyfriend about it and we want to get pregnant. What should I do?"

Elizabeth takes Lourdes's hand. "I know that living with cancer is hard. You are doing well. There are many things to consider . . . "

Discuss the following:

1. What bioethical dilemma exists in Lourdes's situation? In your opinion, is Lourdes's choice to become pregnant an ethical one?
2. How do deeply held beliefs and attitudes about parenthood and the role of women in our society have an impact on the patient's decision? How could these beliefs have an impact on the health care team's response to Lourdes?
3. What is Elizabeth's best therapeutic response to Lourdes? What medical issues should the health care team consider if Lourdes becomes pregnant?
4. What is the role of the medical assistant in this situation?

SELF-ASSESSMENT

A. List and describe the five Ps of ethical power and identify how you are able to demonstrate the five Ps in your own life.

(1) _____

_____

_____

_____

(2) _____

_____

_____

_____

(3) _____

_____

_____

_____

(4) _____

_____

_____

_____

(5) _____

_____

_____

_____

B. List the eight questions adapted from Stephen Covey's book that can be used as guidelines for making ethical decisions. Identify how your life fits into these guidelines and where/if you are striving to do better.

(1) _____

_____

(2) _____

_____

(3) _____

_____

(4) _____

_____

(5) _____

_____

(6) _____

_____

(7) _____

_____

(8) _____

_____

CHAPTER POST-TEST

This is similar to the Pre-Test. Perform this test without looking at the book. This is just to see how well you have understood and can recall the information presented in this chapter after you have studied it and completed the workbook exercises. You will not be graded on this portion (other than the grade you give yourself), but this is an excellent preparation for your instructor's test. You may use this Post-Test to determine what areas you need to study more. Justify any "false" answers.

1. Doing what is right is called ethical behavior. (T or F)
2. Ethical issues dealing with human life is called bioethics. (T or F)
3. The physician and medical assistant have ethical responsibilities to report suspected abuse. (T or F)
4. A physician may refuse to treat an HIV-positive patient. (T or F)
5. Whether to perform abortions is a choice each physician and medical assistant can make for themselves. (T or F)

CERTIFICATION CRITERIA CHECKLIST

As you go through your education and training, keep in mind the national certification examination that you will take when you graduate. Each chapter of the textbook and workbook covers a different section of the examination criteria. To keep track of your preparation for the certification examination, turn to the back of this workbook and highlight the following CMA, RMA, or CMAS certification examination criteria (if you have already highlighted them from a previous chapter, put a check mark by the criteria):

CMA
D. Professionalism
    1. Displaying professional attitude
    3. Performing within ethical boundaries
    4. Maintaining confidentiality
F. Medicolegal Guidelines & Requirements
    2. Legislation
    5. Physician–patient relationship

RMA
I. General Medical Assisting Knowledge
    E. Medical Ethics
        1. Principles of medical ethics and ethical conduct

CMAS
1. Medical Assisting Foundation
    • Professionalism
    • Legal and ethical considerations
4. Medical Records Management
    • Confidentiality
8. Medical Office Management
    • Risk management and quality assurance

EVALUATION OF CHAPTER KNOWLEDGE

Skills	Student Self-Evaluation		
	Good	Average	Poor
I am open to exploring and building a strong personal ethic.	____	____	____
I have respect for the morals and values of others.	____	____	____
I understand the need to maintain confidentiality of patient records.	____	____	____
I understand and can apply the AAMA Code of Ethics and Creed to the ambulatory care setting.	____	____	____
I recognize the seven standards of conduct outlined by the AMA for physicians.	____	____	____
I recognize common ethical issues across the life span.	____	____	____
I can identify sensitive bioethical dilemmas.	____	____	____
I will uphold the honor, integrity, and professionalism of the medical assisting profession.	____	____	____

CHAPTER 9

Emergency Procedures and First Aid

Visit the American Red Cross Web site for information on cardiopulmonary resuscitation (CPR) guidelines at: http://www.redcross.org.

CHAPTER PRE-TEST

Perform this test without looking at the book. This is just to see how well you have understood and can recall the information in this chapter after you have read it, but before you have completed the workbook exercises. You will not be graded on this portion (other than the grade you give yourself). Justify any "false" answers.

1. Of the following, which is the most important in an emergency?
   a. if the patient has medical insurance
   b. if the patient is HIV-positive
   c. if the patient is taking any medication
   d. if the patient is breathing

2. The ABCs of CPR are:
   a. attitude, breathing, circulation
   b. airway, bleeding, circulation
   c. airway, breathing, circulation
   d. airway, bleeding, cardiac

3. As a medical assistant, you are required to perform CPR and first aid in an emergency. (T or F)

4. A first-degree burn is the worst because it has damaged deeper tissues. (T or F)

5. Whenever a person has a penetrating object imbedded in his or her body, it is important that you remove it as soon as possible so you can treat the wound. (T or F)

INTRODUCTION

Medical assistants may encounter emergency situations and should be familiar with the many types of potential emergencies that may occur both within the ambulatory care setting and outside of the office environment. In the ambulatory care setting, primarily designed to see patients in nonemergency situations, a physician is usually available to provide emergency care. The ambulatory care setting also contains medical equipment and supplies to address various emergency situations. The medical assistant, however, is often the first health care professional to interact with an emergency patient. The physician–employer will establish policies and procedures for emergency situations in an emergency policies and procedures manual for the ambulatory care setting that all employees, including medical assistants, will follow in emergency situations. The manual should be reviewed at regularly scheduled staff meetings. Emergency care is provided under the physician's instruction and according to the guidelines established in the emergency policies and procedures manual. Medical assistants must develop the essential skills of triaging emergency situations, that is, of recognizing emergency situations and correctly identifying the measures that must be taken to provide immediate care. As with any health care professional, medical assistants should provide emergency care only within the scope of their knowledge and training. Certified medical assistants (CMAs) must be provider care level CPR and First Aid certified from either American Red Cross, American Heart, American Safety and Health Institute, or National Safety Council.

PERFORMANCE OBJECTIVES

After successful completion of this chapter you will be able to recognize, prepare for, and respond to emergencies. You will understand the precautions you should take when rendering first aid or CPR. You will be able to identify different types of open or closed wounds, burns, and injuries to muscles, bones, and joints, and will be able to describe heat- and cold-related illnesses, the different kinds of shock, and the symptoms of a heart attack or stroke. You also will be able to perform the abdominal thrust maneuver, rescue breathing, and CPR. You should be able to obtain provider level competency to become certified in CPR and First Aid. *The following statements are related to your learning objectives for this chapter. Fill in the blanks in the following paragraphs with the appropriate term(s).*

It is important that medical assistants are able to (1) _____,

(2) _____, and (3) _____ to emergencies. Certain

(4) _____ should be taken when rendering CPR and first aid, including

assessing that the scene of the emergency is (5) _____. Wounds may

be categorized as either (6) _____ or (7) _____. Burns are categorized

according to their severity. A (8) _____ -degree burn is usually superficial, a

(9) _____ -degree burn has burned through partial thickness of the skin, and a

(10) _____ -degree burn has damaged the full thickness of the skin. Bone fractures

are categorized according to the style of break, whether the bone has broken through the skin, as

in a (11) _____ fracture, whether the bone has been twisted, as seen in

a (12) _____ fracture, and if the bone has fragmented into several pieces, as in a

(13) _____ fracture. The main difference between a strain and a sprain is that a (14) _____ involves a joint, whereas a (15) _____ is a muscle injury. Heat stroke differs from heat exhaustion in that the person experiencing heat (16) _____ will be sweating. Although both heat stroke and heat exhaustion are serious, heat (17) _____ is critical. (18) _____ _____ is a method of giving the victim your oxygen until they can breathe on their own. (19) _____ is a method of helping a person who is choking, and (20) _____ is the treatment of choice when a person's heart has stopped beating.

VOCABULARY BUILDER

Find the key vocabulary below that are misspelled; circle them, and then correctly spell them in the spaces provided.

anaphalaxis

automated external defibillator

cardiapulmonary resusitation

cardioversion

crepidation

explicit

fracture

Heimlich manuever

hypothermia

occlusion

syncopy

_____   _____   _____

_____   _____   _____

Word Game

Find the words in the grid. Pick them out from left to right, top line to bottom line. Words can go horizontally, vertically, and diagonally in all eight directions. When you are finished, the first few unused letters in the grid will spell out a hidden message.

```
B E A W A R E E O F Y O U R O W N S A F
E T T R I A G E U Y A S S Y O U C A G Y
R E F O R O T S H C P E R S I N A S R C
N E M E R G P E N R S C Y X X M D T E N
S Y T M L I P R A Z Z E C Q L E Y R E E
Q P H V R Q P I B K K C R H T L S A N G
D C L A R C N W S G Y V O U D M H I S R
N F L I T C O R K Y N G N M Q K O N T E
E D V G N U R V K R N I M X P Q C K I M
G K V N N T V R W I M C H Q X O K T C E
A K L D H M N L S M R D O T W L U D K M
D L S F L M Z S O R J I J P A B T N L Z
N H T T Z C E C P T J A D R E E R D D L
A V G D P R C B R N T T Y Q P R R L K D
B W L R D N D F M Y R S Z T Q K R B D Z
C A R D I A C G W C P R G N I D E E L B
V G E R U T C A R F H I J L N V T Q N N
N O I S S E R P E D L F N K Z J M F M W
F A N A P H Y L A X I S W L N H B N T N
Z D T H Y P O T H E R M I A K T H B K P
```

anaphylaxis	depression	shock
bandage	dressing	spiral
bleeding	emergency	splint
breathing	first aid	sprain
cardiac	fracture	strain
comminuted	greenstick	syncope
compound	hypothermia	triage
CPR	rescue	wounds

Identify each of the following correct vocabulary terms as an emergency condition (EC), an emergency or first aid procedure performed by health care professionals (EP), emergency equipment (EQ), or an emergency service provided to assist in emergency situations (ES).

A. _____ A. first aid

_____ B. triage

_____ C. syncope

_____ D. shock

_____ E. wounds

_____ F. crash tray or cart

_____ G. Heimlich maneuver

_____ H. occlusion

_____ I. universal emergency medical identification symbol and card

_____ J. hypothermia

_____ K. Standard Precautions

_____ L. CPR

_____ M. sprain

_____ N. emergency medical services (EMS)

_____ O. fractures

_____ P. splints

_____ Q. strain

_____ R. rescue breathing

B. *Match each key vocabulary term given in part A with its definition listed below.*

_____ 1. A break in a bone. There are several types, but all are classified as open or closed.

_____ 2. A tray or portable cart that contains medications and supplies needed for emergency and first aid procedures.

_____ 3. An injury to the soft tissue between joints that involves the tearing of muscles or tendons and occurs often in the neck, back, or thigh muscles.

_____ 4. A break in the skin or underlying tissues, categorized as open or closed.

_____ 5. Closure of a passage.

_____ 6. An injury to a joint, often an ankle, knee, or wrist, that involves a tearing of the ligaments. Most are minor and heal quickly; others are more severe, include swelling, and may not heal properly if the patient continues to put stress on the affected joint.

_____ 7. A local network of police, fire, and medical personnel trained to respond to emergency situations. In most communities, the system is activated by calling 911.

_____ 8. Abdominal thrusts designed to overcome breathing difficulties in patients who are choking.

_____ 9. Identification sometimes carried by individuals to identify any health problems they might have.

_____ 10. Any device used to immobilize a body part. Often used by EMS personnel.

_____ 11. An extremely dangerous cold-related condition that can result in death if the individual does not receive care and if the progression of the condition is not reversed. Symptoms include shivering, cold skin, and confusion.

_____ 12. Fainting.

_____ 13. The immediate care provided to persons who are suddenly ill or injured, typically followed by more comprehensive care and treatment.

_____ 14. A condition in which the circulatory system is not providing enough blood to all parts of the body, causing the body's organs to fail to function properly.

_____15. The combination of rescue breathing and chest compressions performed by a trained individual on a patient experiencing cardiac arrest.

_____16. To assess patients' conditions and prioritize the need for care.

_____17. Performed in individuals in respiratory arrest, this is a mouth-to-mouth (using appropriate protective equipment) or mouth-to-nose procedure that provides oxygen to the patient until emergency personnel arrive.

_____18. Guidelines issued by the Centers for Disease Control and Prevention (CDC) in 1996 that combine many of the basic principles of Universal Precautions and body substance isolation techniques. These augmented 1996 guidelines represent the new requirements for infection control measures and are intended to protect health care professionals, patients, and visitors.

LEARNING REVIEW

1. Keen observation skills are necessary to recognize potential emergency situations; medical assistants rely on sight, hearing, and even smell, and they must be acutely sensitive to unusual behaviors. To identify the nature of the emergency and respond effectively, what five things must the medical assistant do to triage, or assess, the patient's situation?

(1) _____

(2) _____

(3) _____

(4) _____

(5) _____

2. In an urgent care setting, two or more patients may present with emergency symptoms. The order in which emergency patients will receive care depends on the health care professionals' abilities to triage patients' symptoms to determine who needs care most urgently.

   The following five patients present simultaneously on New Year's Eve at Inner City Health Care, an urgent care center. Office manager Walter Seals, CMA, is working the evening shift with Dr. Mark Woo. In what order will Walter and Mark triage the priority of treatment?

   Number the patients 1 through 5 to correspond to the urgency of their conditions, one being most critical. For each patient, list the emergency conditions he or she is suffering from, in order of severity, and name the emergency procedures the health care team will initiate to treat the patient.

   A. A patient presents with a gunshot wound to the leg that is bleeding severely. The patient is conscious but his pupils are dilated and he is unable to answer simple questions put to him by Walter and Dr. Woo. He cradles his right arm and will not let anyone touch it, although there is no immediate evidence of an open wound to the arm.

   Urgency of Condition: _____

   _____

   _____

   _____

B. An elderly man, brought in by his grandson, describes debilitating chest pains and nausea after eating a large family dinner. The man is a regular patient of Dr. Ray Reynolds, another physician at Inner City Health Care. The patient's medical record indicates that he has a hiatal hernia, slipped disks, high blood pressure, and mild angina. His vital signs are within a normal range for his general physical condition. The man is walking and speaking with moderate distress and is extremely anxious.

Urgency of Condition: _____

_____

_____

C. A young woman presents with her boyfriend. She appears to have multiple abrasions on her right palm and knee, with damage to the right knee and ankle joints sustained after a fall on in-line skates. Both joints are swollen and painful. She received the skates as a Christmas gift from her boyfriend.

Urgency of Condition: _____

_____

_____

D. A man in his mid-30s presents with the cotton tip of a cotton swab stuck in his ear canal. The tip became lodged in his ear while he was showering and dressing for a New Year's Eve party. Although the man feels a dull consistent pain in the ear, he says he has no trouble hearing. The outside of the ear appears normal, and the man appears annoyed but not distressed.

Urgency of Condition: _____

_____

_____

E. A young woman presents with a group of friends, all college students, with an eye injury sustained by a champagne cork. The cork, which had a metal covering over its tip, hit the patient's eye; the students bring the cork with them. The young woman's eye is red and tearing, and she is experiencing severe pain in the eye.

Urgency of Condition: _____

_____

_____

3. In administering emergency care in the ambulatory care setting, medical assistants and all health care professionals must follow Standard Precautions to protect themselves, their patients, and visitors. What five infection control measures can health care professionals follow to greatly reduce the risk for transmitting infectious disease when providing emergency care?

(1) _____

(2) _____

(3) _____

(4) _____

(5) _____

4. The medical crash cart or tray contains emergency or first aid supplies and medications health care professionals commonly use in treating emergencies. Using a medical encyclopedia or reference such as the *Physician's Desk Reference* (PDR), describe the following emergency medications and identify potential uses for each. Remember that only a physician can order medications or treatment.

A. Lidocaine _____

_____

_____

B. Verapamil _____

_____

_____

C. Atropine _____

_____

_____

D. Insulin _____

_____

_____

E. Nitroglycerin _____

_____

_____

F. Marcaine _____

_____

_____

G. Diphenhydramine _____

_____

_____

H. Diazepam _____

_____

_____

5. Shock requires immediate medical attention. Progressive shock can reach an irreversible point and is life threatening. Shock occurs when the circulatory system is not providing enough blood to all parts of the body, causing the body's organs to function improperly.

For each of the patient symptoms or conditions below, identify the type of shock that is most likely.

_____ A. Patient suffers heart attack

_____ B. Patient experiences severe infection after colon surgery

_____ C. Patient experiences syncope after witnessing a traumatic event

_____ D. Patient experiences reaction to food allergy

_____   E. Choking patient has extreme difficulty breathing

_____   F. Diabetic patient lapses into a coma

_____   G. Patient has serious head trauma

_____   H. Accident victim experiences extreme loss of blood

6. A common procedure for treating closed wounds is to RICE them. What do the letters of this acronym stand for?

R_____   I_____   C_____   E_____

7. *Match each type of open wound to its defining characteristics.*

A. incision

B. puncture

C. laceration

D. avulsion

E. abrasion

_____ 1. A wound that pierces and penetrates the skin. This wound may appear insignificant, but actually can go quite deep.

_____ 2. These wounds commonly occur at exposed body parts such as the fingers, toes, and nose. Tissue is torn off and wounds may bleed profusely.

_____ 3. A wound that results from a sharp object such as a scalpel blade.

_____ 4. A painful wound that involves nerve endings. The epidermal layer of the skin is scraped away.

_____ 5. A wound that results in a jagged tear of body tissues and may contain debris.

8. For each type of wound, describe proper emergency concerns, care, and treatment.

Incision _____

_____

_____

Puncture _____

_____

_____

Laceration _____

_____

_____

Avulsion _____

_____

_____

Abrasion _____

_____

_____

9. Name three sources other than heat that can cause burns. For each, describe the proper emergency concerns, care, and treatment.

   (1) _____

   _____

   _____

   _____

   (2) _____

   _____

   _____

   _____

   (3) _____

   _____

   _____

   _____

10. Musculoskeletal injuries, or injuries to muscles, bones, and joints, can be difficult to triage, especially for closed fractures. List five assessment techniques health care professionals can use to determine the seriousness of musculoskeletal injuries.

    (1) _____

    (2) _____

    (3) _____

    (4) _____

    (5) _____

11. For each set of symptoms that follows, identify the most likely emergency condition and describe emergency concerns, care, and treatment.

    _____ A. Off-color, cold skin with a waxy appearance

    _____

    _____

    _____ B. Hives, itching, lightheadedness

    _____

    _____

    _____ C. Cold, clammy skin; profuse sweating; abdominal cramps; headache; general weakness

    _____

    _____

    _____ D. Lightheadedness, weakness, nausea, unsteadiness

    _____

    _____

_____   E. Moist, pale skin; drooling; lack of appetite; diplopia; full pulse

_____

_____   F. Numbness in face, arm, and leg on one side of body; slurred speech; nausea and vomiting

_____

_____   G. Fever, convulsions, clenched teeth

_____

_____   H. Cold, clammy skin; anxiety; dilated pupils; weak pulse; rigid boardlike abdomen postsurgery for hysterectomy

_____

_____

12. Identify the method of entry into the body for each of the following poisons:

_____   A. carbon monoxide

_____   B. insect stingers

_____   C. chemical pesticides used in the garden

_____   D. spoiled food

_____   E. poison oak

_____   F. cleaning fluid fumes

Emergency Procedure 1

13. Lenore McDonell, a wheelchair-bound woman in her early 30s, experiences a serious laceration to the right arm sustained from a fall while performing an independent transfer from the examination table to her wheelchair. Joe Guerrero, CMA, assists Dr. Winston Lewis in administering emergency care.

   A. What Standard Precautions must the health care professionals follow before administering emergency treatment?

   _____

   _____

   B. Joe and Dr. Lewis attempt to control Lenore's bleeding by applying a dressing and pressing firmly.

   (1) When the bleeding does not stop, what two actions should the health care professionals perform?

   (a) _____

   (b) _____

(2) In the unlikely event that bleeding continues, what piece of medical equipment will the health care team use in substitution of a tourniquet? Why is this alternative equipment effective and widely used today?

_____

_____

_____

_____

C. The bleeding stops, and Joe applies a pressure bandage over the dressing.

(1) This patient is prone to fractures, and a radiograph will need to be taken. What is the next emergency procedure Dr. Lewis will perform? Why is this procedure necessary, and what equipment will the physician and medical assistant require?

_____

_____

_____

(2) Before applying a sling, what do the health care professionals check to be sure that the medical equipment used has not been too tightly applied?

_____

_____

D. What Standard Precautions will the health care team follow after the emergency treatment of the patient is successfully completed?

_____

_____

_____

E. What information will the health care team include in documenting the procedure for the patient's medical record?

_____

_____

_____

_____

Emergency Procedure 2

14. New patient Grace Fisher comes to the offices of Drs. Lewis and King for a well-baby visit for infant Joseph Michael. In the reception area, the baby is fussy; Grace picks him up and holds him at her chest, rocking and gently patting the baby's back. Suddenly, the baby's face becomes red; he begins to cough and wheeze. When the baby does not quickly resume normal breathing, Ellen Armstrong, CMA, alerts Dr. King over the office intercom. As Ellen takes the baby from a bewildered and frightened Grace to begin rescue breathing in a nearby

empty examination room, she motions to coworker Joe Guerrero, CMA, to accompany them to attend to the mother's needs.

A. What four steps will Ellen perform to initiate rescue breathing?

(1) _____

(2) _____

(3) _____

(4) _____

B. Ellen checks for a pulse at the brachial artery. The pulse is present but the baby seems to have increased difficulty breathing. What sequence of actions will Ellen follow next? How long should Ellen continue this sequence?

_____

_____

_____

C. After 3 minutes, the baby is still conscious and has a pulse but is no longer able to cough, cry, or breathe. Dr. King has joined Grace and Ellen in the examination room.

(1) What procedure does Dr. King initiate at this time?

_____

(2) What four steps does Dr. King follow to perform this procedure?

(a) _____

_____

(b) _____

_____

(c) _____

_____

(d) _____

_____

(3) How long will Dr. King continue this procedure?

_____

D. The infant, Joseph Michael, loses consciousness. Grace becomes hysterical.

(1) As she shakes the infant to check for consciousness, Dr. King gives what two instructions to Joe?

(a) _____

(b) _____

(2) Dr. King begins to administer what procedure? How long will Dr. King administer this procedure? What happens if the baby loses a pulse?

_____

_____

E. On the second set of back blows and thrusts after the baby loses consciousness, Dr. King sweeps a bead out of the baby's mouth. Joseph Michael begins to cough and cry. A bead from Grace's sweater had come loose and lodged in the baby's trachea. "We've caught this just in time," Dr. King announces to a grateful and relieved mother.

What follow-up procedures will the health care team initiate?

_____

_____

_____

F. What information will the health care team include in documenting the procedure in the infant's medical record? In Grace's medical record?

(1) *Joseph Michael Fisher:*

_____

_____

_____

_____

(2) *Grace Fisher:*

_____

_____

_____

_____

Emergency Procedure 3

15. Edith Leonard, a frail widow in her early 70s, participates in the knitting club at the local senior center. As she knits, Edith becomes restless and begins to rub her chest and massage her jaw. Her breathing becomes shallow. Bruce Goldman, CMA, who volunteers at the senior center, remembers Edith as a patient at Inner City Health Care, where he works. When Edith slumps in her chair, Bruce rushes over.

A. When Bruce calls Edith's name, she nods her head. However, Edith seems to have extreme difficulty breathing, and her face is contorted with pain. What is Bruce's first action?

_____

B. Edith is no longer breathing. What procedure should Bruce initiate? What steps does Bruce follow in performing the procedure?

_____

_____

_____

_____

C. Edith is still not breathing and no pulse is present.

   (1) What procedure does Bruce initiate?

   _____

   _____

   (2) What is the correct method to administer chest compressions?

   _____

   _____

   (3) How many slow breaths will Bruce administer after completing the chest compressions?

   _____

   _____

   (4) How many times will Bruce repeat the sequence of chest compressions and rescue breathing before again checking Edith's pulse?

   _____

   _____

D. Under what four conditions is it acceptable for Bruce to stop administering this technique of chest compressions and rescue breathing?

   (1) _____
   (2) _____
   (3) _____
   (4) _____

E. After 10 minutes, EMS personnel arrive and transport Edith to a local hospital.

   (1) What Standard pPrecautions will Bruce practice at the senior center after EMS personnel have transported the patient from the scene of the emergency?

   _____

   _____

   (2) What supplies and equipment would the medical assistant have used if this emergency had taken place in an ambulatory care setting?

   _____

   _____

16. Shock that occurs as a result of overwhelming emotional factors such as fear, anger, or grief is called:

   a. neurogenic

   b. psychogenic

   c. anaphylactic

   d. septic

17. The type of burn that may occur resulting in an entrance and exit burn wound area is:
    a. chemical
    b. electrical
    c. solar radiation

18. In burn depth classifications, third-degree burns are also called:
    a. superficial
    b. full thickness
    c. partial thickness

19. The type of fracture often caused by falling on an outstretched hand that involves the distal end of the radius is called:
    a. greenstick
    b. spiral
    c. colles
    d. implicated

20. Jaw and left shoulder pain; a rapid, weak pulse; excessive perspiration; and cold, clammy skin may be symptomatic of:
    a. seizure
    b. heart attack
    c. stroke
    d. sepsis

CERTIFICATION REVIEW

These questions are designed to mimic the certification examinations. You can use these questions like a small "Certification Examination Study Guide," but this is not meant to take the place of the more extensive study guides. Use this portion to determine in what areas to concentrate your efforts when studying for the certification examination. Justify any "false" answers.

1. Which of the following is not an appropriate treatment for hypothermia?
   a. Give the victim warm liquids to drink.
   b. Remove any wet clothing.
   c. Rub the victim's skin vigorously to increase circulation.
   d. Use warm water to warm the person if possible.

2. A diabetic emergency should be treated with sugar. (T or F)

3. In anaphylactic shock, the patient will:
   a. feel a constriction in his or her throat and chest
   b. have difficulty breathing
   c. have swelling and tingling of the lips and tongue
   d. all of the above

4. When performing CPR, the breaths and chest compressions should be at a rate of

    a. 12 to 5

    b. 5 to 12

    c. 15 to 5

    d. 2 to 15

CASE STUDY

Mary O'Keefe calls Dr. King's office in a panic. Ellen Armstrong, CMA, answers the telephone. "Oh my God, help me. I need Dr. King."

    "This is Ellen Armstrong, CMA. Who is this calling and what is the situation?"

    "It's my baby, oh God, get Dr. King."

    "Dr. King is unavailable, but we can help you. Now, tell me your name."

    "It's Mary O'Keefe. Help me, I think my baby is dead."

    "Are you at home?"

    "Yes."

    "Good. Tell me what's happened."

    "My son Chris pried the plug off an outlet and he's electrocuted himself!" Mary cries. "He's just lying there. I'm so scared; if I touch him will I electrocute myself? Oh my God, my baby, my baby. What should I do?"

    Ellen, who has been writing the details on a piece of paper motions to Joe Guerrero, another CMA in the office, and hands him her notes. Joe immediately accesses the O'Keefe's address from the patient database and uses another telephone line to call EMS with the nature of the emergency situation and directions to the O'Keefe's residence. Meanwhile, Ellen remains on the line with Mary. Dr. King is on rounds at the hospital this morning and will not be in the office for at least another hour.

    "Mary, we're calling EMS, and they will be there as soon as possible. In the meantime, I'm going to need you to focus and answer my questions. Okay?"

Discuss the following:

1. What steps does the medical assistant take to triage the emergency situation?
2. What questions should Ellen ask Mary regarding the emergency situation? Based on Mary's answers, what instructions should Ellen give Mary to begin emergency treatment?
3. What should the medical assistant do after EMS arrives and takes over emergency care? What follow-up procedures are necessary?

SELF-ASSESSMENT

1. A. *On a scale of 1 to 5, rate your personal comfort in regard to the following emergency situations medical assistants may find themselves involved with in an ambulatory or urgent care setting.*

1. Extremely uncomfortable	4. Comfortable
2. Uncomfortable	5. Very comfortable
3. Somewhat comfortable	

    _____ Assisting in treatment of patients with injuries clearly sustained by an act of violence or abuse

    _____ Performing the Heimlich maneuver on an unconscious person

    _____ Administering CPR to a child

_____ Administering back blows and thrusts to a conscious infant

_____ Performing rescue breathing on someone who has poor personal hygiene

_____ Bandaging the open wound of an HIV-infected person

_____ Caring for a person experiencing a seizure

_____ Administering care to a patient who faints after venipuncture

_____ Administering care to a patient in extreme pain

_____ Administering care to a patient who is verbally abusive or uncooperative

B.   *On a scale of 1 to 5, rate your level of agreement with the statements that follow.*

1. Never

2. Occasionally

3. Sometimes

4. Most of the time

5. All of the time

_____ Life-threatening emergencies frighten me.

_____ I respond well under pressure.

_____ I am bothered by the sight of blood.

_____ I lose my temper easily, becoming openly frustrated and angry.

_____ I become frustrated and overwhelmed by feelings of helplessness in emergency situations.

_____ I remain calm and clearheaded in emergency situations.

_____ I forget about myself completely and focus on the emergency victim.

_____ I am concerned about administering care in emergency situations in which danger to myself may exist when giving such care.

_____ I am comfortable speaking to the family or friends of emergency victims.

CHAPTER POST-TEST

This test is similar to the Pre-Test. Perform this test without looking at the book. This is just to see how well you have understood and can recall the information presented in this chapter after you have studied it and completed the workbook exercises. You will not be graded on this portion (other than the grade you give yourself), but this is an excellent preparation for your instructor's test. You may use this Post-Test to determine what areas you need to study more. Justify any "false" answers.

1. Of the following, which is the most important in an emergency?

   a. if the patient has medical insurance

   b. if the patient is HIV-positive

   c. if the patient is taking any medication

   d. if the patient is breathing

2. In ABCs of CPR are:

   a. attitude, breathing, circulation

   b. airway, bleeding, circulation

   c. airway, breathing, circulation

   d. airway, bleeding, cardiac

3. As a medical assistant, you are required to perform CPR and first aid in an emergency. (T or F)

4. A first-degree burn is the worst because it has damaged deeper tissues. (T or F)

5. Whenever a penetrating object has been imbedded in a person's body, it is important that you remove it as soon as possible so you can treat the wound. (T or F)

CERTIFICATION CRITERIA CHECKLIST

As you go through your education and training, keep in mind the national certification examination that you will take when you graduate. Each chapter of the textbook and workbook covers a different section of the examination criteria. To keep track of your preparation for the certification examination, turn to the back of this workbook and highlight the following CMA, RMA, or CMAS certification examination criteria (if you have already highlighted them from a previous chapter, put a check mark by the criteria).

CMA
T. Patient Preparation and Assisting the Physician
    1. Performing telephone and in-person screening
X. Emergencies
    1. Preplanned action
    2. Assessment and triage
Y. First Aid
    1. Establishing and maintaining an airway
    2. Identifying and responding to (first aid)
    3. Signs and symptoms
    4. Management (first aid)

RMA
I. General Medical Assisting Knowledge
   A. Anatomy and Physiology
      1. Body systems: Identify the structure and function of
      2. Disorders and diseases: Identify and define various

CMAS
2. Basic Clinical Medical Office Assisting
   • Medical office emergencies

COMPETENCY ASSESSMENT

Procedure 9-1 Control of Bleeding

Performance Objectives: To control bleeding caused by an open wound. Perform this objective within 15 minutes with a minimum score of 30 points.

Supplies/Equipment: Sterile dressings, sterile gloves, mask, eye protection, a gown, biohazard waste container

Charting/Documentation: Enter appropriate documentation/charting in the box.

_____

_____

_____

_____

_____

Instructor's/Evaluator's Comments and Suggestions:

_____

_____

_____

_____

_____

_____

_____

SKILLS CHECKLIST Procedure 9-1: Control of Bleeding

Name _____

Date _____

No.	Skill	Check #1 20 pts ea	Check #2 10 pts ea	Check #3 5 pts ea	Notes
1	Wash hands and gather equipment quickly.				
2	Apply gloves and other PPE; eye mask, gown if splashing likely.				
3	Apply pressure bandages and apply pressure for 10 minutes. If bleeding continues, elevate arm above heart. If continues, press adjacent artery against bone.				
4	Dispose of waste in biohazard container.				
5	Wash hands.				
6	Document procedure.				
Student's Total Points					
Points Possible		120	60	30	
Final Score (Student's Total Points / Possible Points)					

	Notes
Start time:	
End time:	
Total time: (15 min goal)	

COMPETENCY ASSESSMENT

Procedure 9-2 Applying an Arm Splint

Performance Objectives: To immobilize the area above and below the injured part of the arm to reduce pain and prevent further injury. Perform this objective within 15 minutes with a minimum score of 30 points.

Supplies/Equipment: Thin piece of rigid board and gauze roller bandage

Charting/Documentation: Enter appropriate documentation/charting in the box.

_____

_____

_____

_____

Instructor's/Evaluator's Comments and Suggestions:

_____

_____

_____

_____

_____

_____

SKILLS CHECKLIST Procedure 9-2: Applying an Arm Splint

Name _____

Date _____

No.	Skill	Check #1 20 pts ea	Check #2 10 pts ea	Check #3 5 pts ea	Notes
1	Place a padded splint under the injured area.				
2	Hold the splint in place with roller gauze.				
3	Check circulation (note color and temperature of skin and nails, and check pulse).				
4	Apply sling to keep arm elevated.				
5	Wash hands.				
6	Document procedure.				
	Student's Total Points				
	Points Possible	120	60	30	
	Final Score (Student's Total Points / Possible Points)				

	Notes
Start time:	
End time:	
Total time: (15 min goal)	

COMPETENCY ASSESSMENT

Procedure 9-3 Abdominal Thrusts for a Conscious Adult

Performance Objectives: To open a blocked airway. Perform this objective within 15 minutes with a minimum score of 25 points.

Supplies/Equipment: None.

Charting/Documentation: Enter appropriate documentation/charting in the box.

_____

_____

_____

_____

Instructor's/Evaluator's Comments and Suggestions:

_____

_____

_____

_____

_____

_____

SKILLS CHECKLIST Procedure 9-3: Abdominal Thrusts for a Conscious Adult

Name _____

Date _____

No.	Skill	Check #1 20 pts ea	Check #2 10 pts ea	Check #3 5 pts ea	Notes
1	Place thumb side of fist against the middle of the abdomen above the umbilicus and below the xiphoid process.				
2	Grasp the fist with the free hand and give quick upward thrusts.				
3	Repeat until the patient coughs up the object. If the patient loses consciousness, perform abdominal thrusts for unconscious adult.				
4	Wash hands.				
5	Document procedure.				
Student's Total Points					
Points Possible		100	50	25	
Final Score (Student's Total Points / Possible Points)					

	Notes
Start time:	
End time:	
Total time: (15 min goal)	

COMPETENCY ASSESSMENT

Procedure 9-4 Abdominal Thrusts for an Unconscious Adult or Child

Performance Objectives: To open a blocked airway on an unconscious victim. Perform this objective within 15 minutes with a minimum score of 60 points.

Supplies/Equipment: Gloves, a resuscitation mouthpiece, biohazard waste receptacle

Charting/Documentation: Enter appropriate documentation/charting in the box.

_____

_____

_____

_____

Instructor's/Evaluator's Comments and Suggestions:

_____

_____

_____

_____

_____

SKILLS CHECKLIST Procedure 9-4: Abdominal Thrusts for an Unconscious Adult or Child

Name _____

Date _____

No.	Skill	Check #1 20 pts ea	Check #2 10 pts ea	Check #3 5 pts ea	Notes
1	Appoint someone to call emergency services.				
2	Apply gloves.				
3	Lie patient on back and tilt patient's head back.				
4	Open victim's mouth and look for foreign object, then position resuscitation.				
5	Give breaths.				
6	If air will not go in, retilt head and try again. If air will not go in, place heel of the hand against the abdomen and the umbilicus and below the xiphoid process of the sternum.				
7	Kneel astride the patient's thighs and give five abdominal thrusts.				
8	Lift the jaw and sweep out the mouth.				
9	Tilt the head back, lift the chin, and give breaths again. Continue giving breaths and thrusts, sweeping the mouth until breaths go in.				
10	Dispose of waste in biohazard waste receptacle.				
11	Wash hands.				
12	Document procedure.				
Student's Total Points					
Points Possible		240	120	60	
Final Score (Student's Total Points / Possible Points)					

	Notes
Start time:	
End time:	
Total time: (15 min goal)	

COMPETENCY ASSESSMENT

Procedure 9-5 Abdominal Thrusts for a Conscious Child

Performance Objectives: To open a blocked airway. Perform this objective within 15 minutes with a minimum score of 20 points.

Supplies/Equipment: None.

Charting/Documentation: Enter appropriate documentation/charting in the box.

_____

_____

_____

_____

Instructor's/Evaluator's Comments and Suggestions:

_____

_____

_____

_____

_____

_____

SKILLS CHECKLIST Procedure 9-5: Abdominal Thrusts for a Conscious Child

Name _____

Date _____

No.	Skill	Check #1 20 pts ea	Check #2 10 pts ea	Check #3 5 pts ea	Notes
1	Place thumb side of fist against the middle of the umbilicus and below the xiphoid process.				
2	Grasp the fist with the free hand and give quick upward thrusts. Repeat until the object is expelled or until the victim loses consciousness.				
3	Wash hands.				
4	Document procedure.				
Student's Total Points					
Points Possible		80	40	20	
Final Score (Student's Total Points / Possible Points)					

	Notes
Start time:	
End time:	
Total time: (15 min goal)	

COMPETENCY ASSESSMENT

Procedure 9-6 Back Blows and Chest Thrusts for a Conscious Infant Who Is Choking

Performance Objectives: To open a blocked airway and assist a conscious infant who is choking. Perform this objective within 15 minutes with a minimum score of 30 points.

Supplies/Equipment: None.

Charting/Documentation: Enter appropriate documentation/charting in the box.

_____

_____

_____

_____

Instructor's/Evaluator's Comments and Suggestions:

_____

_____

_____

_____

_____

_____

SKILLS CHECKLIST Procedure 9-6: Back Blows and Chest Thrusts for a Conscious Infant Who Is Choking

Name _____

Date _____

No.	Skill	Check #1 20 pts ea	Check #2 10 pts ea	Check #3 5 pts ea	Notes
1	With infant facedown on the forearms, give five back blows between the infant's shoulder blade with the heel of the hand.				
2	Position infant faceup on the forearm.				
3	Give five chest thrusts on about the center of the breastbone.				
4	Look in infant's mouth for the object and repeat back blows and chest thrusts, looking for the object until the infant can breathe on his or her own. If the infant loses consciousness, activate EMS, then use back blows and chest thrust techniques for unconscious infant.				
5	Wash hands.				
6	Document procedure.				
Student's Total Points					
Points Possible		120	60	30	
Final Score (Student's Total Points / Possible Points)					

	Notes
Start time:	
End time:	
Total time: (15 min goal)	

COMPETENCY ASSESSMENT

Procedure 9-7 Back Blows and Chest Thrusts for an Unconscious Infant

Performance Objectives: To open a blocked airway by delivering back blows and chest thrusts for an unconscious infant. Perform this objective within 15 minutes with a minimum score of 85 points.

Supplies/Equipment: Gloves, resuscitation mouthpiece

Charting/Documentation: Enter appropriate documentation/charting in the box.

_____

_____

_____

_____

Instructor's/Evaluator's Comments and Suggestions:

_____

_____

_____

_____

_____

SKILLS CHECKLIST Procedure 9-7: Back Blows and Chest Thrusts for an Unconscious Infant

Name _____

Date _____

No.	Skill	Check #1 20 pts ea	Check #2 10 pts ea	Check #3 5 pts ea	Notes
1	Appoint someone to call emergency services.				
2	Don gloves.				
3	Tap the infant gently to check for consciousness.				
4	Gently tilt back the infant's head.				
5	Apply resuscitation mouthpiece.				
6	Listen and watch for breathing.				
7	Give two breaths, covering the infant's nose and mouth.				
8	If air does not go in, retilt head and make another attempt.				
9	If breaths still do not go in, position the infant facedown on the forearms.				
10	Give back blows with the heel of the hand between the shoulder blades.				
11	Position the infant faceup on the forearms.				
12	Give five chest thrusts on about the center of the breastbone.				
13	Lift the jaw and tongue to check for objects, sweeping it out.				
14	Tilt the head back and give breaths again.				
15	Repeat breaths, back blows, and chest thrusts, and check for objects until the infant is breathing on his or her own.				
16	Wash hands.				
17	Document procedure.				
Student's Total Points					
Points Possible		340	170	85	
Final Score (Student's Total Points / Possible Points)					

	Notes
Start time:	
End time:	
Total time: (15 min goal)	

COMPETENCY ASSESSMENT
Procedure 9-8 Rescue Breathing for Adults

Performance Objectives: To respond to a breathing emergency. Perform this objective within 15 minutes with a minimum score of 60 points.

Supplies/Equipment: Gloves, resuscitation mouthpiece, biohazard waste receptacle

Charting/Documentation: Enter appropriate documentation/charting in the box.

_____

_____

_____

_____

_____

Instructor's/Evaluator's Comments and Suggestions:

_____

_____

_____

_____

_____

_____

SKILLS CHECKLIST Procedure 9-8: Rescue Breathing for Adults

Name _____

Date _____

No.	Skill	Check #1 20 pts ea	Check #2 10 pts ea	Check #3 5 pts ea	Notes
1	Appoint someone to call emergency services.				
2	Don gloves.				
3	Shout "Are you all right?"				
4	Tilt head back and lift chin; position resuscitation mouthpiece and pinch the nose closed.				
5	Give two slow breaths into the patient, turn face to the side, listen, and watch for air return.				
6	Check for pulse on carotid attery.				
7	If pulse is present but the victim is not breathing, give 1 slow breath every 5 seconds for 1 minute.				
8	Recheck pulse and breathing status every minute.				
9	Continue rescue breathing as long as pulse is present and the victim is not breathing. Continue breathing until breathing is restored or someone else takes over.				
10	Disposes of waste in the biohazard container.				
11	Wash hands.				
12	Document procedure.				
Student's Total Points					
Points Possible		240	120	60	
Final Score (Student's Total Points / Possible Points)					

	Notes
Start time:	
End time:	
Total time: (15 min goal)	

COMPETENCY ASSESSMENT

Procedure 9-9 Rescue Breathing for Children

Performance Objectives: To respond to a breathing emergency involving a child. Perform this objective within 15 minutes with a minimum score of 65 points.

Supplies/Equipment: Gloves, resuscitation mouthpiece, biohazard waste receptacle

Charting/Documentation: Enter appropriate documentation/charting in the box.

_____

_____

_____

_____

Instructor's/Evaluator's Comments and Suggestions:

_____

_____

_____

_____

_____

_____

SKILLS CHECKLIST Procedure 9-9: Rescue Breathing for Children

Name _____

Date _____

No.	Skill	Check #1 20 pts ea	Check #2 10 pts ea	Check #3 5 pts ea	Notes
1	Appoints someone to call emergency services				
2	Don gloves.				
3	Position resuscitation mouthpiece.				
4	Tilt head back and lift chin, pinch nose closed, and give two short breaths.				
5	If air does not go in, retilt head and breathe again.				
6	Check for pulse on carotid attery.				
7	If pulse is present but the victim is not breathing, give 1 slow breath every 3 seconds for 1 minute.				
8	Recheck pulse and breathing status every minute.				
9	Continue rescue breathing as long as pulse is present and the victim is not breathing. Continue breathing until breathing is restored or someone else takes over.				
10	Wash hands.				
11	Document procedure.				
Student's Total Points					
Points Possible		260	130	65	
Final Score (Student's Total Points / Possible Points)					

	Notes
Start time:	
End time:	
Total time: (15 min goal)	

COMPETENCY ASSESSMENT

Procedure 9-10 Rescue Breathing for Infants

Performance Objectives: To restore breathing to an infant. Perform this objective within 15 minutes with a minimum score of 55 points.

Supplies/Equipment: Gloves, resuscitation mouthpiece, biohazard waste receptacle

Charting/Documentation: Enter appropriate documentation/charting in the box.

_____

_____

_____

_____

Instructor's/Evaluator's Comments and Suggestions:

_____

_____

_____

_____

_____

_____

SKILLS CHECKLIST Procedure 9-10: Rescue Breathing for Infants

Name _____

Date _____

No.	Skill	Check #1 20 pts ea	Check #2 10 pts ea	Check #3 5 pts ea	Notes
1	Appoint someone to call emergency services.				
2	Don gloves and resuscitation mouthpiece.				
3	Tilt head back.				
4	Seal lips tightly around infant's nose and mouth.				
5	Give two slow breaths into the infant until the chest rises.				
6	Check for pulse on brachial artery.				
7	If pulse is present but the victim is not breathing, give 1 slow breath every 3 seconds for 1 minute.				
8	Recheck pulse and breathing status every minute.				
9	Continue rescue breathing as long as pulse is present and the victim is not breathing. Continue breathing until breathing is restored or someone else takes over.				
10	Wash hands.				
11	Document procedure.				
Student's Total Points					
Points Possible		220	110	55	
Final Score (Student's Total Points / Possible Points)					

	Notes
Start time:	
End time:	
Total time: (15 min goal)	

COMPETENCY ASSESSMENT
Procedure 9-11 CPR for Adults

Performance Objectives: To restore breathing and cardiac activity in an emergency. Perform this objective within 15 minutes with a minimum score of 55 points.

Supplies/Equipment: Gloves, resuscitation mouthpiece, biohazard waste receptacle

Charting/Documentation: Enter appropriate documentation/charting in the box.

_____

_____

_____

_____

Instructor's/Evaluator's Comments and Suggestions:

_____

_____

_____

_____

_____

SKILLS CHECKLIST Procedure 9-11: CPR for Adults

Name _____

Date _____

No.	Skill	Check #1 20 pts ea	Check #2 10 pts ea	Check #3 5 pts ea	Notes
1	Ask "Are you okay, are you okay?" If no response, appoint someone to call emergency services.				
2	Don gloves and resuscitation mouthpiece.				
3	Tilt head back and lift chin.				
4	Look, listen, and feel for breathing for 10–15 seconds. If the patient is not breathing, keep the airway open, pinch the nose, insert mouthpiece, and give two breaths.				
5	Check pulse at the carotid artery for 10–15 seconds; if the patient does not have a pulse, start chest compressions.				
6	After locating the area on the abdomen, 2 inches above the xiphoid, position the shoulders over the hands and compress the chest 15 times.				
7	Give two slow breaths, pinching the nose closed.				
8	Do 3 more sets of 15 compressions and two breaths.				
9	Check the pulse and breathing for 10–15 seconds.				
10	If there is no pulse, continue sets of 15 compressions to 2 breaths.				
11	Disposes of waste in biohazard container.				
Student's Total Points					
Points Possible		220	110	55	
Final Score (Student's Total Points / Possible Points)					
		Notes			
Start time:					
End time:					
Total time: (15 min goal)					

COMPETENCY ASSESSMENT
Procedure 9-12 CPR for Children

Performance Objectives: To respond to a cardiac arrest emergency involving a child. Perform this objective within 15 minutes with a minimum score of 60 points.

Supplies/Equipment: Gloves, resuscitation mouthpiece

Charting/Documentation: Enter appropriate documentation/charting in the box.

_____

_____

_____

_____

Instructor's/Evaluator's Comments and Suggestions:

_____

_____

_____

_____

_____

_____

SKILLS CHECKLIST Procedure 9-12: CPR for Children

Name _____

Date _____

No.	Skill	Check #1 20 pts ea	Check #2 10 pts ea	Check #3 5 pts ea	Notes
1	Tap child to check for consciousness level; if no response, appoint someone to call emergency services.				
2	Don gloves and resuscitation mouthpiece.				
3	Tilt head back, look, listen, and feel for breathing. If there is no breathing, give two slow breaths.				
4	Check carotid artery.				
5	Locate one hand on the breastbone and the other hand on the forehead to maintain an open airway. Using the heel of one hand only, position shoulders over the patient's chest and compress the chest five times.				
6	Give one slow breath while pinching the nose closed.				
7	Repeat cycles of 5 compressions and 1 breath for 1 minute.				
8	Check pulse and breathing for about 5–10 seconds.				
9	If there is no pulse, continue sets of five compressions and one breath.				
10	Recheck the pulse and breathing every few minutes.				
11	Wash hands.				
12	Document procedure.				
Student's Total Points					
Points Possible		240	120	60	
Final Score (Student's Total Points / Possible Points)					

	Notes
Start time:	
End time:	
Total time: (15 min goal)	

COMPETENCY ASSESSMENT

Procedure 9-13 CPR for Infants

Performance Objectives: To restore the heartbeat in a cardiac arrest emergency involving an infant. Perform this objective within 15 minutes with a minimum score of 65 points.

Supplies/Equipment: Gloves, resuscitation mouthpiece

Charting/Documentation: Enter appropriate documentation/charting in the box.

_____

_____

_____

_____

Instructor's/Evaluator's Comments and Suggestions:

_____

_____

_____

_____

_____

_____

SKILLS CHECKLIST Procedure 9-13: CPR for Infants

Name _____

Date _____

No.	Skill	Check #1 20 pts ea	Check #2 10 pts ea	Check #3 5 pts ea	Notes
1	Tap child to check for consciousness level; if no response, appoint someone to call emergency services.				
2	Don gloves and resuscitation mouthpiece.				
3	Tilt head back, look, listen, and feel for breathing. If there is no breathing, give two slow breaths.				
4	Check brachial artery for pulse for 5–10 seconds.				
5	Find finger position on the center of sternum.				
6	Compress the infant's chest five times about 0.5–0.75 inch.				
7	Give one slow breath.				
8	Repeats cycle of 5 compressions and 1 breath for 1 minute.				
9	Recheck brachial pulse and breathing for 5–10 seconds.				
10	If there is no pulse, continue cycles for five compressions and one breath.				
11	Rechecks pulse and breathing every few minutes.				
12	Wash hands.				
13	Document procedure.				
	Student's Total Points				
	Points Possible	260	130	65	
	Final Score (Student's Total Points / Possible Points)				

	Notes
Start time:	
End time:	
Total time: (15 min goal)	

EVALUATION OF CHAPTER KNOWLEDGE

Skills	Student Self-Evaluation		
	Good	Average	Poor
I recognize emergency situations.	⎯⎯	⎯⎯	⎯⎯
I understand the need for emergency preparation and the function of emergency medical services (EMS).	⎯⎯	⎯⎯	⎯⎯
I possess the ability to triage emergency cases in person and over the telephone.	⎯⎯	⎯⎯	⎯⎯
I understand legal and health considerations of emergency caregiving.	⎯⎯	⎯⎯	⎯⎯
I understand the necessity of providing emergency care only within the scope of training and knowledge.	⎯⎯	⎯⎯	⎯⎯
I can assemble a medical crash tray or cart.	⎯⎯	⎯⎯	⎯⎯
I understand the use of Standard Precautions in emergency situations.	⎯⎯	⎯⎯	⎯⎯
I can identify signs and symptoms of shock, types of shock, and treatment of shock.	⎯⎯	⎯⎯	⎯⎯
I can identify classification and care of wounds.	⎯⎯	⎯⎯	⎯⎯
I can identify dressings, bandages, and their applications.	⎯⎯	⎯⎯	⎯⎯
I can identify first-, second-, and third-degree burns and burn care.	⎯⎯	⎯⎯	⎯⎯
I can identify musculoskeletal injuries, including types of fractures and strategies for care.	⎯⎯	⎯⎯	⎯⎯
I can identify heat- and cold-related illnesses and priorities for care.	⎯⎯	⎯⎯	⎯⎯
I understand how poisons enter the body.	⎯⎯	⎯⎯	⎯⎯
I can identify sudden illnesses such as syncope, seizures, diabetes, and hemorrhage.	⎯⎯	⎯⎯	⎯⎯
I recognize cerebral vascular accident (CVA) and priorities for immediate emergency care.	⎯⎯	⎯⎯	⎯⎯
I recognize heart attack and priorities for immediate emergency care.	⎯⎯	⎯⎯	⎯⎯
I can identify and name steps for performing these emergency procedures:			
Control of bleeding	⎯⎯	⎯⎯	⎯⎯
Applying a splint	⎯⎯	⎯⎯	⎯⎯
Abdominal thrusts	⎯⎯	⎯⎯	⎯⎯
Rescue breathing	⎯⎯	⎯⎯	⎯⎯
Cardiopulmonary resuscitation (CPR)	⎯⎯	⎯⎯	⎯⎯

CHAPTER 10

Creating the Facility Environment

CHAPTER PRE-TEST

Perform this test without looking at the book. This is just to see how well you have understood and can recall the information in this chapter after you have read it, but before you have completed the workbook exercises. You will not be graded on this portion (other than the grade you give yourself). Justify any "false" answers.

1. A reception area should:
   a. be comfortable
   b. be clean and uncluttered
   c. contain current reading materials for all ages
   d. all of the above

2. It is considerate, but not required, to provide at least one handicapped patient parking space. (T or F)

3. Keeping the reception area clean is a responsibility of:
   a. the receptionist
   b. the bookkeeper
   c. the medical assistant
   d. the office manger
   e. all of the above

INTRODUCTION

Medical assistants are generally employed in ambulatory care settings, such as the medical office or clinic. The physical environment of the health care facility is an important contributing factor to patient comfort. Effective facility design and layout can also increase efficiency and boost the medical facility's functional utility. Medical assistants recognize that maintaining a professional, welcoming environment for patient care promotes health and increases patient confidence in the physician and in the entire health care team. Complying with the Americans with Disabilities Act (ADA) also ensures that the physically challenged have equal access to care.

PERFORMANCE OBJECTIVES

After successful completion of this chapter you will be able to describe a comfortable and efficient reception area, list and describe the specific items that should be present, and describe the arrangement of the furnishings, the role of Health Insurance Portability and Accountability Act (HIPAA) on the reception area, and the effect your reception area has on your patients. You will be able to discuss the requirement of the ADA for your office entrance and space. You will be able to describe the characteristics of a good medical receptionist and cite the procedures to follow when the patient's appointment is delayed. You will also know how to open and close the office. *The following statements are related to your learning objectives for this chapter. Fill in the blanks in the following paragraph with the appropriate term(s).*

The reception area should make the patient feel (1) _____, secure, and comfortable. Proper seating should be available with adequate (2) _____ for reading. The furnishings should be able to accommodate at least (3) _____ hour's patients per physician, assuming that one friend or relative will accompany each patient. If the clinic sees children or expects that patients will bring children, a special (4) _____ area should be set aside with appropriate (5) _____ and books. The receptionist should have the (6) _____ and (7) _____ to handle many situations without getting upset. He or she must be willing to assist patients whenever necessary and keep the schedule flowing smoothly. Although keeping the reception area neat and clean is probably the responsibility of the (8) _____, all employees should contribute by noticing and correcting any untidy or unclean situation. When opening the facility in the morning, the reception area should be checked, the patient (9) _____ should be prepared if not done so the day before, and the answering (10) _____ should be checked for messages. When closing the facility, all equipment should be checked to make sure it is (11) _____, doors and (12) _____ should be secured, all (13) _____ material should be locked away or covered, and the (14) _____ cash should be locked away.

VOCABULARY BUILDER

Find the words below that are misspelled; circle them, and then correctly spell them in the spaces provided. Then insert vocabulary terms from the list that best fit into the descriptive sentences below.

accessibility	characteristic	infomatics
accountibility	enviroment	receptionist

_____   _____   _____

1. _____ Information available through the Internet or other electronic format

2. _____ The physical space of the reception area

3. _____ A typical or distinguishing quality

4. _____ The medical assistant who greets the patient and begins the patient visit process: this person may also answer the phones

5. _____ Being ultimately responsible

6. _____ Being readily reachable

Word Game

Find the words in the grid. Pick them out from left to right, top line to bottom line. Words can go horizontally, vertically, and diagonally in all eight directions. When you are finished, the first few unused letters in the grid will spell out a hidden message.

```
L  S  C  I  T  A  M  R  O  F  N  I  O  O  P  E
K  E  A  T  Y  F  A  C  I  L  I  T  Y  L  S  N
O  U  L  R  R  E  C  E  P  G  T  I  A  O  C  V
N  A  R  B  E  A  A  S  N  A  A  Y  P  G  I  I
A  D  E  L  A  Y  S  I  T  C  I  T  E  N  T  R
N  T  W  O  U  T  D  L  C  D  S  V  I  I  S  O
D  E  L  W  A  A  R  E  I  I  T  .  F  T  I  N
T  E  F  I  E  A  S  O  N  K  T  K  V  I  R  M
J  J  S  R  G  S  P  O  F  G  P  B  T  V  E  E
F  N  N  I  I  H  I  I  N  M  T  Y  T  N  T  N
R  N  Z  B  G  T  T  I  H  K  O  M  O  I  C  T
L  D  L  H  P  N  M  I  Z  Z  R  C  Y  A  A  V
K  E  V  E  L  L  H  B  N  Z  N  Q  S  D  R  K
N  T  C  W  A  G  P  L  Q  G  M  Z  M  A  A  L
R  E  L  C  B  G  N  I  M  O  C  L  E  W  H  V
R  K  M  N  R  F  U  R  N  I  T  U  R  E  C  G
```

accessible	environment	play
ADA	facility	reading
calming	furniture	receptionist
characteristics	HIPAA	toys
comfortable	informatics	welcoming
delays	inviting	
design	lighting	

LEARNING REVIEW

1. A. What is the purpose of the ADA?

   _____

   _____

   _____

   _____

   B. When creating the facility environment, why is accessibility a major consideration?

   _____

   _____

   _____

   _____

   C. Name four ways an ambulatory care setting can accommodate the physically challenged.

   (1) _____

   (2) _____

   (3) _____

   (4) _____

2. The physical office environment can contribute to the patient's sense of confidence and comfort, or it can be viewed by the patient as intimidating or anxiety producing. For each office area below, describe why the area could be perceived by patients as a frightening place. What can be done to make each area a more comforting environment for patients?

   Reception area _____

   _____

   _____

   _____

   Corridors _____

   _____

   _____

   _____

   Examination rooms _____

   _____

   _____

   _____

3. Health care professionals should strive to empower the patient with as much control and dignity as possible. For each of the following situations listed, identify strategies that health care professionals can use to respect the patient's dignity and lessen the sense of disproportion between health care providers and the patient.

A. Bill Schwartz is referred to a dermatologist by Dr. Ray Reynolds for examination of a suspicious mole on his calf. The dermatologist tells Bill that a full-body inspection will need to be done to ensure that no other areas of the skin are affected. Bill must appear disrobed in front of the dermatologist and medical assistant, who are both female.

_____

_____

_____

B. Martin Gordon, diagnosed with prostate cancer, begins a series of radiation treatments. At the radiation clinic, he is required to disrobe from the waist down and put on a hospital gown. While waiting for access to the treatment room, Martin must sit in a common area with other patients, male and female, who are also waiting for radiation treatments.

_____

_____

_____

C. Ellen Armstrong, CMA, places a Holter monitor on patient Charles Williams. After the Holter monitor is in place, Charles has several questions about the patient activity diary that he would prefer to discuss with Dr. Winston Lewis.

_____

_____

_____

4. The medical receptionist, often a medical assistant with other duties to perform as well, is the person who sets the social climate for the interchange between the patient and the health care team. A friendly, reassuring demeanor and an ability to triage situations are essential skills. For each situation listed, what is the best action or response of the medical receptionist?

A. A patient with intense stomach pain doubles over, and then bolts up to the reception desk, saying, "I'm going to throw up."

_____

_____

_____

_____

B. When presented with a bill, the patient exclaims, "I can't pay for all of this now! Every time I come here it seems like the doctor bill goes up a hundred dollars."

_____

_____

_____

_____

C. A patient is looking for the correct exit from the examination area to the waiting area and makes a wrong turn into the receptionist's area. He asks, "Where do I go?"

_____

_____

D. A patient new to an HMO plan does not realize that a separate referral form is needed for a follow-up visit with the gastroenterologist one week after a colonoscopy test has been performed. She says, "I drove an hour to get to this appointment. No one told me I needed another form."

5. Identify at least four things to be done in the reception area to accommodate children.
   (1) _____
   (2) _____
   (3) _____
   (4) _____

6. A. Create a checklist of five activities to perform on opening a medical facility.
   (1) _____
   (2) _____
   (3) _____
   (4) _____
   (5) _____

   B. Create a checklist of five activities to perform on closing a medical facility.
   (1) _____
   (2) _____
   (3) _____
   (4) _____
   (5) _____

7. Making facilities and equipment available to all users is called:
   a. maintenance
   b. accessibility
   c. promotion
   d. standardization

8. HIPAA requires that clinic facilities:
   a. have adequate corridors and bathrooms to accommodate wheelchair patients
   b. place a receptionist in an area seen and heard by all patients

c. protect the confidentiality of patients checking in at the reception desk

d. provide space for children in the clinic

9. The primary goal of maintaining a comfortable environment in which patient care is given is to:

a. feed anxiety

b. aggravate illness

c. promote health

d. stimulate the senses

10. Space planners suggest:

a. that the reception area accommodate at least 2 hours' patients per physician

b. that the reception area can accommodate a friend or relative who might accompany each patient

c. that there be 2.5 seats in the reception area for each examination room

d. only b and c

11. Any drugs kept in the office that are identified as controlled substances must always be kept:

a. in the refrigerator

b. in a locked, secure cabinet

c. in the physician's desk drawer

d. in the receptionist's desk drawer

CERTIFICATION REVIEW

These questions are designed to mimic the certification examinations. You can use these questions like a small "Certification Examination Study Guide," but this is not meant to take the place of the more extensive study guides. Use this portion to determine where to concentrate your efforts when studying for the certification examination.

1. HIPAA has changed the way we organize our entrance and reception areas in the following way:

a. Patients must be able to see the receptionist at all times.

b. Patients must have adequate parking.

c. Patients must not be able to see or hear confidential information about other patients.

d. The magazines must be current.

2. ADA states that:

a. Patients must not know the names and diagnoses of other patients.

b. Handicapped patients must have access to all patient areas with reasonable accommodations.

c. Visually impaired patients must have adequate lighting and contrast for better viewing.

d. An interpreter must be present with any non–English-speaking patient.

3. Patient safety within the reception area is accomplished by:
   a. providing chairs that are sturdy and in good repair
   b. containing wires and cords and keeping them out of reach
   c. attaching rugs to the flooring without loose edges
   d. containing toys within a designated play area
   e. all of the above

CASE STUDY

Lydia Renzi, a deaf woman with some residual hearing, is a patient of Dr. Angie Esposito's at Inner City Health Care. Lydia is fluent in American Sign Language (ASL) and usually wears a hearing aid when she is away from home.

Lydia calls to make her appointment at Inner City Health Care using a telecommunications device for the deaf (TDD) and the services of a government-funded relay operator. Although Lydia often chooses not to be accompanied by an interpreter, Inner City Health Care always provides the option to supply the services of a qualified professional sign language interpreter in compliance with the ADA. When Lydia arrives at Inner City Health Care with a high fever and a suspected case of the flu, the staff accommodates Lydia's special needs in several simple ways. Remembering that deaf people rely on visual images to receive and to convey messages, Liz Corbin, CMA, always faces Lydia directly so that the patient can see her facial expressions and lip movements. Liz holds eye contact with Lydia and does not break it until she is sure that Lydia understands her message and has time to think and respond. Special care is taken to provide Lydia with written instructions for prescriptions and for following through on home care.

Discuss the following:
1. What are the special communication needs of the hearing-impaired patient in the ambulatory care setting?
2. How can the medical assistant's actions make a direct impact on the quality of care given to hearing-impaired patients?
3. Suppose that Lydia is an elderly woman who is embarrassed and sensitive about her hearing loss and will not admit that she has trouble hearing others. How might the medical assistant accommodate the special needs of this patient?

SELF-ASSESSMENT

1. Visualize your last visit to a medical facility. Was the reception area clean, tidy, welcoming, and comfortable? What would you do to improve it?

_____

_____

_____

_____

2. List at least three things you would add to any reception area to make it even more accommodating. Think of items not mentioned in the textbook.

_____

_____

_____

_____

CHAPTER POST-TEST

This is similar to the Pre-Test. Perform this test without looking at the book. This is just to see how well you have understood and can recall the information presented in this chapter after you have studied it and completed the workbook exercises. You will not be graded on this portion (other than the grade you give yourself), but this is an excellent preparation for your instructor's test. You may use this Post-Test to determine what areas you need to study more. Justify any "false" answers.

1. A receptioning area should:
   a. be comfortable, clean, and uncluttered
   b. contain current reading materials for all ages
   c. have adequate lighting for reading
   d. contain accommodations for patients with disabilities
   e. all of the above

2. It is required to provide at least one handicapped patient parking space. (T or F)

3. Keeping the reception area clean is a responsibility of:
   a. the receptionist
   b. the bookkeeper
   c. the medical assistant
   d. the office manger
   e. all employees

CERTIFICATION CRITERIA CHECKLIST

As you go through your education and training, keep in mind the national certification examination that you will take when you graduate. Each chapter of the textbook and workbook covers a different section of the examination criteria. To keep track of your preparation for the certification examination, turn to the back of this workbook and highlight the following CMA, RMA, or CMAS certification examination criteria (if you have already highlighted them from a previous chapter, put a check mark by the criteria):

CMA
F. Medicolegal Guidelines & Requirements
    2. Legislation
    3. Documentation/reporting
O. Managing the Office
    1. Maintaining the physical plant

RMA
II. Administrative Medical Assisting
    C. Medical Receptionist/Secretarial/Clerical
        2. Reception
        5. Records and chart management
        9. Office safety

CMAS
3. Medical Office Clerical Assisting
    • Reception
4. Medical Records Management
    • Systems
    • Confidentiality

EVALUATION OF CHAPTER KNOWLEDGE

Skills	Student Self-Evaluation		
	Good	Average	Poor
I can identify tasks in opening and closing the facility.	____	____	____
I recognize the importance of the medical receptionist.	____	____	____
I can relate the physical environment of the facility to the patient's care and comfort.	____	____	____
I can relate the physical environment of the facility to optimal functionality and efficiency.	____	____	____
I know how to safeguard patient privacy.	____	____	____
I understand the purpose of the ADA and can describe methods of compliance.	____	____	____
I am able to empathize with the patient experience of the health care facility.	____	____	____

CHAPTER 11

Computers in the Ambulatory Care Setting

CHAPTER PRE-TEST

Perform this test without looking at the book. This is just to see how well you have understood and can recall the information in this chapter after you have read it, but before you have completed the workbook exercises. You will not be graded on this portion (other than the grade you give yourself). Justify any "false" answers.

1. One main advantage of e-mail is:
   a. you have an immediate response
   b. messages are secure
   c. everybody has access
   d. you do not have to play "telephone tag"

2. To ensure that your work in the computer is safe, you should:
   a. use only formatted discs
   b. defragment frequently
   c. use firewalls
   d. backup frequently

3. Circle each of the following that is a computer function:
   a. keeping track of appointments
   b. keeping track of accounts receivable
   c. keeping track of accounts payable
   d. processing insurance claims

4. The "brain" of the computer is called the:
   a. motherboard
   b. math coprocessor

   c. video card

   d. central processing unit (CPU)

5. To prevent unauthorized use of your clinic computers, you should:

   a. keep the computer in a locked cabinet at all times

   b. keep the computer in a locked cabinet at night

   c. assign every employee a password

   d. have only one person on the computer at a time

6. The difference between a spreadsheet and a database is:

   a. Databases keep track of numbers.

   b. Spreadsheets calculate numbers.

   c. Databases organize information.

   d. Spreadsheets organize information.

   e. They are both the same and function the same.

INTRODUCTION

Ambulatory care settings have made the transition from manual to computerized systems. Medical assistants with a knowledge of computer equipment, or hardware, and computer programs, or software, are a strong asset to the medical office. Today, computers are used in complex clinical applications such as assisting in performing sensitive surgeries, diagnosing illnesses, and developing patient treatment strategies. In the ambulatory care setting, physicians purchase computer systems to perform administrative tasks, such as patient data collection, correspondence, reports, billing, and insurance claim filing. Confidentiality of computerized patient records must be strictly maintained. Medical assistants are expected to be able to learn and use office computer applications. Often, medical assistants are involved in researching and implementing computer applications for specific administrative office functions. Medical assisting students are encouraged to explore the potential of computers. Perhaps intimidating at first, with a little experience computers can become user-friendly tools that offer valuable methods for streamlining tasks and increasing efficiency in the ambulatory care setting.

PERFORMANCE OBJECTIVES

After successful completion of this chapter you will be able to define the correct vocabulary terms in this chapter, describe the basic elements of a computer system, identify main types of computers, list examples of input and output devices, explain how computer information can be stored, describe networks, explain the various uses for computers in the medical clinic, explain ergonomics, cite ways to prevent computer viruses, use various computer software applications, and explain how Health Insurance Portability and Accountability Act (HIPAA) regulations can be maintained within a computerized office. You will be able to follow professional behavior while using clinic computers. *The following statements are related to your learning objectives for this chapter. Fill in the blanks in the following paragraph with the appropriate term(s).*

The four fundamental elements of a computer are (1) _____,

(2) _____, (3) _____, and

(4) _____. Four main types of computers are

(5)_____ , (6) _____ ,

(7) _____ , and (8) _____ .

Two examples of commonly used input devices are (9) _____

and (10) _____ . Two examples of output devices are

(11) _____ and (12) _____ .

Three common ways to store computer information are (13) _____ ,

(14) _____ , and (15) _____ .

Networks might best be described as an (16) _____ connection of

two or more computers for the purpose of sharing information. Hardwired networks are referred

to as (17) _____ . Wireless systems are capable of a much (18) <u>(more or less)</u> rapid

rate of data transmission than the hard-wired systems. Hard-wired systems are (19) <u>(more or less)</u>

secure from hacking or other unauthorized access. One way of protecting the clinic computer from

damage from an outside source is to install (20) _____

software and keep it updated. HIPAA privacy rules require that no (21) _____

persons be allowed access to private medical and personal information. One way to accomplish

this when patient information is stored on computers is to use (22) _____ .

VOCABULARY BUILDER

A. *Find the words below that are misspelled; circle them, and then correctly spell them in the spaces provided. Then insert the correct vocabulary terms from the list that best fit the descriptions below.*

A. erganomics
B. hardware
C. Internet
D. maneframe computer
E. microcomputer
F. minicomputer

G. modom
H. personal computer
I. RAM
J. supercomputer
K. system

_____   _____   _____

_____ 1. A device used by a computer to communicate to a remote computer through phone lines

_____ 2. The scientific study of work and space, including factors that influence workers' productivity and that affect workers' health

_____ 3. A large computer system capable of processing massive volumes of data

_____ 4. A personal, or desktop, computer

_____ 5. Acronym for random access memory, a type of computer memory that can be written to and read from

_____ 6. The physical equipment used by the computer system to process data

_____ 7. Larger than a microcomputer and smaller than a mainframe

_____ 8. A worldwide computer network available via modem

_____ 9. The fastest, largest, and most expensive computers currently being manufactured

_____ 10. Also known as microcomputer

_____ 11. A unit composed of a number of parts that function together to perform a particular task

B. *Find the words below that are misspelled; circle them, and then correctly spell them in the spaces provided. Then insert the correct vocabulary terms from the list that best fit the descriptions below.*

A. applications software
B. bit
C. byte
D. communications software
E. data
F. database managment software
G. documentation
H. electronic mail
I. feilds
J. footers
K. graphics software
L. headers

M. information retieval systems
N. macros
O. merge mail
P. operating system
Q. orphen
R. record
S. software
T. sort
U. spreadsheat software
V. widow
W. word processing software

_____

_____ _____

_____

_____ 1. A page formatting feature that allows the bottom of all pages to be marked consistently with keyed-in data

_____ 2. The raw material; the collection of characters and numbers entered into a computer

_____ 3. A word processing operation designed to produce form letters

_____ 4. Software that provides instructions to the computer hardware and also runs computer programs

_____ 5. Systems that allow electronic access to large databases for the retrieval of information

_____ 6. Related fields, grouped together and organized in the same order

_____ 7. Smallest unit of data a computer can process

_____ 8. Applications software used to create pictorial representations

_____ 9. A frequently used data processing operation that arranges data in a particular sequence or order

_____ 10. In typesetting, a term describing the situation in which a new paragraph begins on the last line of a printed page

_____ 11. Communications that take place online from computer to computer by means of a modem

_____ 12. Equivalent of a computer program or programs

_____ 13. Amount of memory needed to store one character

_____ 14. A page formatting feature that allows the top of a page to be printed with identifying information

_____ 15. A series of keystrokes that have been saved under a separate file name that can be used and inserted repeatedly into a document or documents

_____ 16. Software that performs a specific data processing function

_____ 17. A computer application that allows the user to format and edit documents before printing

_____ 18. A basic data category within the database

_____ 19. Computer applications packages that act as "number crunchers" because of their mathematical processing capabilities

_____ 20. Written material that accompanies purchased software, containing the information necessary for using the software appropriately

_____ 21. Applications software used for the transfer of data from one computer system to another

_____ 22. In typesetting, a term describing the situation in which a line of text that is the end of a paragraph ends on a new page of printed text

_____ 23. Applications software designed for the manipulation of data within a database

LEARNING REVIEW

1. Medical assistants may encounter many types of software in the ambulatory care setting, including scheduling (S); word processing (WP); clinical (C); accounting (A); billing, collecting, and insurance (BCI); and practice management (PM).

   Identify the tasks listed below according to the type of software used to perform them by placing the proper letters in the spaces provided.

   _____ A. inventories and drug supplies   _____ H. check writing

   _____ B. medical records   _____ I. labels and addressing

   _____ C. aging accounts receivable   _____ J. prescription writing

   _____ D. patient reminders   _____ K. payroll

   _____ E. employee vacation records   _____ L. thank you letters

   _____ F. charge slips   _____ M. consultation reports

   _____ G. insurance claim processing   _____ N. treatment plans

2. Computer systems are great assets to any ambulatory care setting in streamlining tasks and increasing productivity. Special steps need to be taken to keep the systems operating at peak efficiency. Name three steps medical assistants should take in the care and handling of computer components.

   (1) _____

   (2) _____

   (3) _____

3. There are six operations that are fundamental to the operation of any computer software. Identify the proper operation in the examples below.

_____ A. Administrative medical assistant Ellen Armstrong, CMA, working in the offices of Drs. Lewis and King, makes adjustments in format and corrects spelling and punctuation errors in a thank you letter the practice sends to new patients.

_____ B. Ellen prepares a hard copy of Martin Gordon's treatment plan for Dr. Winston Lewis.

_____ C. Office manager Marilyn Johnson, CMA, asks Ellen to add columns to the existing drug inventory spreadsheet.

_____ D. Ellen enters data on employee vacation and sick time into the new spreadsheet software.

_____ E. After entering all of the patient addresses into a single file, Ellen makes sure that the file will be retained permanently.

_____ F. On request from Dr. Elizabeth King, Ellen produces the most recent correspondence sent to patient Maria Jover.

4. Word processing is largely concerned with the production of textual material and is an integral part of the ambulatory care setting. Match the following common word processing features with the correct descriptions.

A. multicolumn output   D. sorting
B. macros   E. import and export
C. page formatting   F. block operations

_____ 1. These allow the user to highlight and move text to another position within the document

_____ 2. This refers to the rearrangement of information

_____ 3. Allows users to carry a text file into another applications program

_____ 4. Keystrokes that have been saved separately so the saved keystrokes may be inserted into any document

_____ 5. The arrangement of text on a page in two or more columns

_____ 6. This is used to create a variety of looks for the printed page

5. Spreadsheet software "crunches," or calculates, numbers. Define the following elements of spreadsheet programs.

A. Cell location _____

B. Worksheet _____

C. Values _____

D. Labels _____

Name three tasks for which spreadsheet software is particularly useful.

(1) _____

(2) _____

(3) _____

6. A. Databases or database management systems (DBMS) are built from the concept of data organization. Name four elements that comprise the organization of data.

   (1) _____   (3) _____

   (2) _____   (4) _____

   B. Ellen Armstrong, CMA, is creating a patient database for the offices of Drs. Lewis and King. The office currently maintains information on 1,000 patients. List 10 fields of information the database should contain to track the patients.

   (1) _____

   (2) _____

   (3) _____

   (4) _____

   (5) _____

   (6) _____

   (7) _____

   (8) _____

   (9) _____

   (10) _____

7. The use of computerized databases in the delivery of health care services is becoming an established methodology for patient care. However, the trend toward computerizing medical records and the electronic processing of insurance claims presents challenges in preserving patient confidentiality.

   A. Name the federal legislation that protects against unauthorized access or interception of data communication.

   _____

   B. The _____ has put forth guidelines to follow for the enactment of laws that protect individual privacy and confidentiality.

8. The American Medical Association (AMA) has published computer confidentiality guidelines to assist physicians and computer service organizations in maintaining the confidentiality of information in medical records when that information is stored in computerized databases.

   A. Confidential medical information should be entered into the computer-based patient record only by _____.

B. The person making any additions to the record should be _____.

C. The computerized medical database should be online to the computer terminal only when _____ are being used.

D. Name three security measures that can be used to control access to the computerized database.

(1) _____

(2) _____

(3) _____

9. The monitor or screen that provides a real-time feedback of what is taking place with input data is:

a. data storage

b. data output

c. formatting

d. retrieval

10. Accounting, scheduling, and insurance coding are examples of:

a. application software

b. system software

c. word processing software

d. database management

11. Arrangement of information so that it is concise, easy to read, and in word processing files includes setting margins, line spacing, and tab settings is:

a. editing

b. file creation

c. retrieval

d. formatting

12. One of the health hazards associated with repetitive computer use is:

a. Ménière's disease

b. Bell's palsy

c. carpal tunnel syndrome

d. rheumatoid arthiritis

13. A term used for the precautions taken to prevent persons from hacking into computer systems through the Internet is:

a. dam

b. firewall

c. stonewall

d. retention wall

CERTIFICATION REVIEW

These questions are designed to mimic the certification examinations. You can use these questions like a small "Certification Examination Study Guide," but this is not meant to take the place of the more extensive study guides. Use this portion to determine what areas to concentrate your efforts when studying for the certification examination.

1. A flashing bar that indicates where you are on the computer screen is called the:
   a. scroll bar
   b. cursor
   c. flash bar
   d. input bar

2. A flash drive is a:
   a. memory device
   b. type of software device
   c. a DVD drive
   d. a safety warning

3. Hacker is a term given to:
   a. a computer operator with inconsistent word processing
   b. a computer operator with a very bad cough
   c. a computer that goes off and on for no reason
   d. a person who gets into a computer system without permission

4. RAM stands for:
   a. reality actuated memory
   b. random access memory
   c. right access mouse
   d. retrieval access motherboard

5. Firewalls will prevent:
   a. fires from damaging your information
   b. fires from damaging your computer
   c. damage from spreading from one area of your computer to another
   d. damage from unauthorized access

6. Defragmenting gets rid of:
   a. fragments of information that you do not need anymore
   b. old information no longer needed
   c. empty spaces within your database
   d. fragments of software that you do not use

CASE STUDY

The offices of Drs. Lewis and King recently experienced a pronounced surge in patient load when the physician–employers agreed to accept patients from several HMOs operating in the area. The group practice added two new staff members, co-office manager Shirley Brooks, CMA, and clinical medical assistant Anna Preciado, CMA. To handle the increased load of paperwork, Dr. Winston Lewis asks Shirley to devise a database to identify patient insurance variables. The practice already has a functional database of patient information.

Discuss the following:

1. What strategies will Shirley use to research the proper database software and to determine the desired organization of information within the new patient insurance database?
2. What information will the patient insurance database need to contain to allow for the streamlining of paperwork and claims processing?
3. What will the office manager do when she has completed her research and has devised a plan for assembling the patient insurance database?

SELF-ASSESSMENT

1. How comfortable are you with moving a computer from one area to another and hooking up all the cords, connections, and wires? What do you think you could do to become more comfortable with computer hardware connections. Look at the connections of your computer and its accessory hardware. Is it color coded or marked in some way?

2. How comfortable are you with installing a software program onto a computer? Would you be able to do it by yourself? How about defragmenting? Formatting a disc? Updating virus protection? Next time it is appropriate to perform these actions, ask your technical support person/department to let you watch, or ask a technically experienced person to show you how.

3. Have you explored all the options in your e-mail software system? Set up groups? Set up signatures? Asked for a return reply? Explore the options and set up these actions.

CHAPTER POST-TEST

This is similar to the Pre-Test. Perform this test without looking at the book. This is just to see how well you have understood and can recall the information presented in this chapter after you have studied it and completed the workbook exercises. You will not be graded on this portion (other than the grade you give yourself), but this is an excellent preparation for your instructor's test. You may use this Post-Test to determine what areas you need to study more. Justify any "false" answers.

1. A disadvantage of e-mail is:
   a. you do not have an immediate response
   b. messages are not secure
   c. not everyone has access
   d. all of the above

2. To ensure that your computer information is safe from unauthorized viewing:
   a. use only formatted discs
   b. defragment frequently
   c. use firewalls
   d. backup frequently

3. Which of the following is a not a computer function:
    a. keeping track of appointments
    b. keeping track of accounts receivable
    c. keeping track of accounts payable
    d. processing insurance claims
    e. fixing dinner

4. A circuit board that houses the chips for the CPU, RAM, and ROM is called the:
    a. motherboard
    b. math coprocessor
    c. video card
    d. CPU board

5. To prevent unauthorized use of your clinic's computers, you should:
    a. establish only one person who has access to the computer
    b. keep the computer in a locked cabinet at night
    c. assign every employee a password
    d. have only one person on the computer at a time

6. A database:
    a. keeps track of numbers and other information
    b. calculates numbers
    c. organizes information
    d. functions like a spreadsheet

CERTIFICATION CRITERIA CHECKLIST

As you go through your education and training, keep in mind the national certification examination that you will take when you graduate. Each chapter of the textbook and workbook covers a different section of the examination criteria. To keep track of your preparation for the certification examination, turn to the back of this workbook and highlight the following CMA, RMA, or CMAS certification examination criteria (if you have already highlighted them from a previous chapter, put a check mark by the criteria):

CMA
D. Professionalism
        4.   Maintaining confidentiality
F. Medicolegal Guidelines & Requirements
        2.   Legislation
G. Data Entry
        1.   Keyboard fundamentals and functions
H. Equipment
I.   Computer Concepts

RMA
II. Administrative Medical Assisting
      C. Medical Receptionist/Secretarial/Clerical
            8. Computer applications

CMAS
7. Medical Office Information Processing
- Fundamentals of computing
- Medical office computer applications

COMPETENCY ASSESSMENT

Procedure 11-1 Software Installation

Performance Objectives: To add software to the computer system for later call up and use. Perform this objective within 15 minutes with a minimum score of 15 points for automatic installation and 25 points for manual installation.

Supplies/Equipment: Manual, computer, software program

Charting/Documentation: Enter appropriate documentation/charting in the box.

_____

_____

_____

_____

Instructor's/Evaluator's Comments and Suggestions:

_____

_____

_____

_____

_____

SKILLS CHECKLIST Procedure 11-1: Software Installation

Name _____

Date _____

No.	Skill	Check #1 20 pts ea	Check #2 10 pts ea	Check #3 5 pts ea	Notes
Automatic Installation					
1	Close all open programs.				
2	Insert the CD provided with the program into the CD drive.				
3	Follow the instructions given by the software documentation and the Installation Wizard screens that appear.				
4	At the completion of the program, you will respond to questions appropriately. Example is the registration of the software package.				
Manual Installation					
1	Close all open programs.				
2	Insert CD. Click START, then select RUN from the menu.				
3	Respond to the questions appropriately, such as the name and address of the program you want to run for installation.				
4	Include the letter destination for the drive where the program is located (usually D drive). Common name is: Setup. Example: D:\setup.				
5	Follow onscreen instructions.				
Student's Total Points					
Points Possible (depending on type of installation)		60 or 100	30 or 50	15 or 25	
Final Score (Student's Total Points / Possible Points)					
	Notes				
Start time:					
End time:					
Total time: (15 min goal)					

COMPETENCY ASSESSMENT

Procedure 11-2 Hardware Installation

Performance Objectives: To add hardware to the computer system for later use. Perform this objective within 15 minutes with a minimum score of 25 points for automatic installation and 15 points for manual installation.

Supplies/Equipment: Manual, computer, hardware to be installed

Charting/Documentation: Enter appropriate documentation/charting in the box.

_____

_____

_____

_____

Instructor's/Evaluator's Comments and Suggestions:

_____

_____

_____

_____

_____

SKILLS CHECKLIST Procedure 11-2: Hardware Installation

Name _____

Date _____

No.	Skill	Check #1 20 pts ea	Check #2 10 pts ea	Check #3 5 pts ea	Notes
Using Automatic Initiation from Microsoft Windows® Installation Wizard					
1	Close all open programs.				
2	Answer questions appropriately such as: Manufacturer and Model Number of the hardware				
3	How the hardware is connected to the computer (Via USB, Parallel, or IEEE 1394 cable).				
4	Whether the driver was supplied with the hardware or already registered with Microsoft.				
5	Follow further directions.				
Using Manual Initiation of Microsoft Windows® Installation Wizard					
1	Close all open programs.				
2	Go to START, SETTINGS, CONTROL PANEL, and double click ADD HARDWARE.				
3	Follow onscreen instructions.				
Student's Total Points					
Points Possible (depending on type of installation)		100 or 60	50 or 30	25 or 15	
Final Score (Student's Total Points / Possible Points)					

	Notes
Start time:	
End time:	
Total time: (15 min goal)	

or say the words clearly. Simple terms rather than medical (3) _____

promote mutual understanding rather than confusion or (4) _____.

The use of slang words and expressions is considered unprofessional and disrespectful. When

speaking with a caller who is not (5) _____ in English, it

is helpful to speak slowly and use short sentences. Proper (6) _____ of all

words in a carefully (7) _____ voice will also help people understand what you

are saying, especially non–English-speaking people. Good (8) _____ skills

are of real benefit to a medical assistant when using the telephone and when speaking directly to

patients. The use of (9) _____ _____ can help the sentences make sense

to the patient. Responding with empathy conveys an appreciation for the caller's concerns and

needs. Medical assistants will screen and route calls that come into the medical facility to ensure

that callers speak to the appropriate staff member who can (10) _____

their medical problems. Because complete patient confidentiality is considered a legal and

(11) _____ obligation, medical assistants must not discuss patients

outside of the professional environment or share any patient information with nonmedical

professionals without written patient permission. And, of course, always remember that the

(12) _____ _____ _____ will only protect those medical assistants

who stay within their scope of practice when interacting with patients or the public.

B. *Match the following devices or services listed in Column A with corresponding descriptions in Column B.*

Column A

1. _____ pager

2. _____ answering service

3. _____ cellular phone

4. _____ automated routing unit

5. _____ fax

6. _____ e-mail

Column B

A. Takes calls when the office is closed

B. Sends a message via phone lines to an electronic mailbox located in another person's computer

C. A one-way communication device used to contact staff when away from the office

D. A portable telephone

E. A document sent over telephone lines from one facsimile machine or modem to another

F. A system that allows callers to reach specific people or departments by pressing a specified number on a touch-tone telephone

LEARNING REVIEW

1. Effective telephone communication requires prompt and professional responses from medical assistants. For each of the scenarios listed below, what should the medical assistant say to give the best telephone response?

   A. Karen Ritter, CMA, answers the first call of the morning at Inner City Health Care.

   Medical assistant: _____

   _____

   _____

   B. Patient Nora Fowler calls with a question about medication prescribed for her rheumatoid arthritis and insists on a call back from Dr. Elizabeth King. Dr. King is presently on rounds at the hospital and will not be available until 4:30 PM. Nora's tone of voice indicates that she is distrustful of the medication and of the physician's reliability, and it is clear from the conversation that Nora has discontinued taking her medication.

   Medical assistant: _____

   _____

   _____

   C. While speaking on telephone line 1 with patient Bill Schwartz, who is calling to schedule a physical examination, medical assistant Wanda Slawson receives another call on line 2 from a laboratory with a summary of emergency test results for another patient. Wanda knows Dr. Susan Rice is waiting for the test results.

   Medical assistant: _____

   _____

   _____

   D. Bruce Goldman, CMA, takes a call from patient Juanita Hansen. Juanita is inquiring about a bill and indicating that her insurance carrier, Blue Cross, did not pay the entire fee for her son's last examination, which left her with a balance owed to Inner City Health Care. Office manager Walter Seals is responsible for managing insurance claims and inquiries.

   Medical assistant: _____

   _____

   _____

2. Showing compassion and concern for the well-being of the caller allows both potential and established patients to feel confident about the high quality of care they receive.

   A. Name four reasons why a potential patient will contact an ambulatory care facility by telephone.

   (1) _____

   (2) _____

   (3) _____

   (4) _____

B.   What seven pieces of information should a medical assistant record in the appointment book when scheduling an initial appointment with the physician?

(1) _____   (5) _____

(2) _____   (6) _____

(3) _____   (7) _____

(4) _____

3.   Indicate the calls described below that fall within the scope of practice for a medical assistant (MA) to respond to and the calls that should be directed to the physician (P). For each call handled by a medical assistant, describe the information needed to address the needs of the caller. For each call referred to the physician, give reasons why a physician must handle the call.

_____   A. Insurance questions

_____

_____

_____   B. Scheduling patient testing and office appointments

_____

_____

_____   C. Medical emergencies

_____

_____

_____   D. Requests for prescription refills

_____

_____

_____   E. Complaints about medical care or treatment

_____

_____

_____   F. General information about the practice

_____

_____

_____   G. Poor progress reports from a patient

_____

_____

_____   H. Requests for medications other than prescription refills

_____

_____

_____ I. Medical questions

_____

_____

_____ J. Salespeople

_____

_____

4. Answering services and answering machines are two methods of taking calls after hours. Answering services are staffed by live operators who take messages for the physician and medical practice when the office is closed. Answering machines can also be used for taking the majority of after-hours calls, with a telephone number given in the outgoing message that will connect callers with a live operator in the event of an emergency.

A. Compose an appropriate outgoing message for the offices of Drs. Lewis and King.

_____

_____

_____

_____

B. Each morning, administrative medical assistant Ellen Armstrong is responsible for transcribing messages left on the medical practice's answering machine the evening before. Using the message pad slips in Figure 12-1, transcribe each message completely and appropriately. In the space for "Attachments," list any records, files, or documents that should be attached to the message slip for the recipient's review.

Message 1. "Ellen, this is Anna Preciado. Can you tell [office manager,] Marilyn, that I won't be in tomorrow for the afternoon shift? I've got a 101 degree temperature and bad flu symptoms. Maybe Joe Guerrero can come in to sub for me as the clinical medical assistant; yesterday, he said he might be available if I wasn't feeling well enough to come in. I know Dr. Lewis has several patients scheduled for clinical testing in the afternoon. I'm at 555-6622. Thanks."

Message 2. "This is Heidi from Dr. Kwiczola's office calling for Dr. Lewis. We have a new patient, Marsha Beckman, in our psychiatric practice who is experiencing symptoms of fatigue, anxiety, palpitations, and weight loss. Dr. Kwiczola suspects this patient may be suffering from hyperthyroidism. Dr. Kwiczola will be in the office tomorrow from 2 PM to 7 PM and can be reached at 555-7181."

Message 3. "This is Martin Gordon, a patient of Dr. Lewis's. I need to talk to Shirley Brooks, the office manager who handles insurance. I've got a question about my out-of-pocket maximum."

Message 4. "This is Charles Williams. Dr. Lewis put me on a Holter monitor today. It's about 11 PM. and one of the leads came off. I put it back on, but I'm worried about whether I'll have to do this test again. Can you call me at home before eight at 555-6124 or at the office after nine at 555-8125?"

Message #1

To: _____   Date: _____

From: _____   Time: _____

Telephone #: _____

Message: _____

_____

_____

_____

Initials: _____

Attachments: _____

_____

_____

_____

(a)

Message #2

To: _____   Date: _____

From: _____   Time: _____

Telephone #: _____

Message: _____

_____

_____

_____

Initials: _____

Attachments: _____

_____

_____

_____

(b)

Message #3

To: _____   Date: _____

From: _____   Time: _____

Telephone #: _____

Message: _____

_____

_____

_____

Initials: _____

Attachments: _____

_____

_____

_____

Message #4

To: _____   Date: _____

From: _____   Time: _____

Telephone #: _____

Message: _____

_____

_____

_____

Initials: _____

Attachments: _____

_____

_____

_____

Figure 12-1   **(c)**   **(d)**

5. Medical assistants must observe laws regarding patient confidentiality and the patient's right to privacy.

Indicate which people and under what restrictions a medical assistant may discuss a patient's medical condition or reveal details from the medical record.

Person	Yes, without signed release	No	Yes, with signed release
A. Patient's spouse or family	☐	☐	☐
B. Patient's employer	☐	☐	☐
C. Patient's attorney	☐	☐	☐
D. Another health care provider	☐	☐	☐
E. Insurance carrier or HMOs	☐	☐	☐
F. Referring physician's office	☐	☐	☐
G. Credit bureaus or collection agencies	☐	☐	☐

Person	Yes, without signed release	No	Yes, with signed release
H. Members of the office staff, as necessary for patient care	☐	☐	☐

_____

_____

_____

| I. Patient's insurance carrier | ☐ | ☐ | ☐ |

_____

_____

_____

| J. Other patients | ☐ | ☐ | ☐ |

_____

_____

_____

| K. People outside the office (friends, family, acquaintances of the medical assistant) | ☐ | ☐ | ☐ |

_____

_____

_____

| L. Patient's parent or legal guardian, except concerning issues of birth control, abortion, or sexually transmitted diseases | ☐ | ☐ | ☐ |

_____

_____

_____

6. Many physicians and health care professionals use paging systems. Paging systems allow the medical assistant to alert a physician or other health care professional who is not on-site to call in for an important message. Name and describe four paging system options.

   (1) _____

   _____

   _____

   (2) _____

   _____

   _____

(3) _____

_____

_____

(4) _____

_____

_____

7. The term that best describes speaking clearly and articulating carefully is:

   a. pronunciation

   b. modulation

   c. enunciation

   d. fluency

8. The act of evaluating the urgency of a medical situation and prioritizing treatment is:

   a. screening

   b. referral

   c. triage

   d. etiquette

9. To ensure sensible risk management when making calls, you should protect the patient's privacy at all times; this is referred to as:

   a. confidentiality

   b. jargon

   c. elaboration

   d. screening

10. Many hospitals and ambulatory care settings have telephone systems to manage heavy telephone traffic; these are called:

    a. ARU

    b. CPU

    c. ATT

    d. BLS

11. No call should be left unattended for more than:

    a. 1 minute

    b. 2 minutes

    c. 20–30 seconds

    d. 5 minutes

CERTIFICATION REVIEW

These questions are designed to mimic the certification examinations. You can use these questions like a small "Certification Examination Study Guide," but this is not meant to take the place of the more extensive study guides. Use this portion to determine in what areas to concentrate your efforts when studying for the certification examination.

1. Telephone calls that may be handled by the medical assistant include all but which one of the following?

   a. billing questions

   b. appointment changes

   c. requests for prescription refills

   d. calls from other physicians

2. When a medical assistant is talking to a patient on the telephone and another line rings, what should the medical assistant do?

   a. Put the first call on hold, answer the second call, put that caller on hold, and go back to the first caller to finish up.

   b. Put the first call on hold, answer the second call and handle that issue, then go back to the first caller.

   c. Let the second line ring; it will be picked up by an answering system.

   d. Finish with the first caller, then answer the second line.

3. Which of the following is not a good idea in a medical office?

   a. using a speaker phone to listen to voice messages

   b. speaking quietly on the telephone so other patients cannot hear

   c. using a privacy screen to reduce the chance of being overheard on the telephone

   d. using only e-mail so you will not be overheard

4. After-hours telephone messages are usually directed to:

   a. the physician's home

   b. the medical manager's home

   c. a voice mail system or answering service/machine

   d. an e-mail system

5. When talking to older adult patients on the phone:

   a. If the patient is hearing impaired, speak slower, clearer, and a little louder.

   b. Assume they are senile or at least forgetful and repeat all the information several times.

   c. If the person has difficulty understanding, simplify the information, ask if there are any questions, and try to explain patiently in simple terms.

   d. all of the above

   e. a and c only

6. Health Insurance Portability and Accountability Act (HIPAA) guidelines for telephone communications include:

   a. Determine if the patient has specific instructions on who has been granted privilege to their private medical information.

   b. Determine if the patient has a particular number they want called for confidential communications.

   c. Ask if it is acceptable to leave a message if the patient is not at the number provided.

   d. All of the above.

CASE STUDY

As Inner City Health Care, an urgent care center, continues to grow, increasing both patient load and staff, the existing telephone system consisting of a simple intercom and four telephone lines is no longer sufficient to handle the call volume and allow for full, immediate accessibility for all staff members. Callers are frustrated by the length of time it takes to get through and by long amounts of time spent on hold. Messages are often late in getting properly routed. Administrative medical assistant Karen Ritter suggests to office manager Jane O'Hara that an automated routing unit (ARU) might be more efficient for the growing clinic's needs. At the next regularly scheduled staff meeting, the physician–employers give the go-ahead to research an ARU.

Discuss the following:
1. ARU systems provide several options for callers that identify specific departments or services that callers can be connected with directly. What kinds of caller options might be appropriate for Inner City Health Care?
2. What can be done so emergency patients or hearing-impaired patients can speak automatically to a "live" operator?
3. How can an ARU help staff members receive their calls more efficiently?
4. How can the office manager and medical assistant implement the ARU system with a minimum of disruption to physicians, staff, and patients?

SELF-ASSESSMENT

Discuss the following questions with another classmate or in a small group. During the discussion, consider how different people react in different ways, depending on their personalities, their patience, and their confidence levels. After the discussion, spend a moment in self-reflection to think of ways you can improve your telephone communication skills.

1. Have you ever conversed with someone on the telephone whom you could not understand?

2. Was it his or her language, accent, enunciation, or volume?

3. Would it have been easier to understand him or her if you were face to face with him or her?

4. How did you handle the situation? Did you ask the person to speak louder, slower, or more clearly?

5. How do you think most people would handle a situation in which they could not hear the speaker clearly? Older adults? Non–English speakers? People in pain or very ill?

Of the following telecommunication devices and methods, with which are you familiar and which will you need to learn more about? What do you think is the best way to become more familiar with the devices and methods?

1. e-mail
2. pagers
3. handheld devices
4. multiline phones
5. cellular phones
6. instant messaging
7. fax machines
8. answering services

CHAPTER POST-TEST

This is similar to the Pre-Test. Perform this test without looking at the book. This is just to see how well you have understood and can recall the information presented in this chapter after you have studied it and completed the workbook exercises. You will not be graded on this portion (other than the grade you give yourself), but this is an excellent preparation for your instructor's test. You may use this Post-Test to determine what areas you need to study more. Justify any "false" answers.

1. When transferring a call, it is important to obtain the patient's name and phone number. (T or F)

2. Some patients will become defensive when a firm voice is used on the phone. (T or F)

3. We always have time to ask patients if they can be put on hold. (T or F)

4. When taking a message, be brief but thorough. The patient's name, phone number, questions, best time for a call back, and any other pertinent information are useful. (T or F)

5. Patients should expect confidentiality at all times, even on their home answering machines. (T or F)

6. The physician should be alerted to any angry calls regarding patient care and treatment. (T or F)

CERTIFICATION CRITERIA CHECKLIST

As you go through your education and training, keep in mind the national certification examination that you will take when you graduate. Each chapter of the textbook and workbook covers a different section of the examination criteria. To keep track of your preparation for the certification examination, turn to the back of this workbook and highlight the following CMA, RMA, or CMAS certification examination criteria (if you have already highlighted them from a previous chapter, put a check mark by the criteria):

CMA
E. Communication
    1. Adapting communication to an individual's ability to understand
    4. Professional communication and behavior
    5. Evaluating and understanding communication
    7. Receiving, organizing, prioritizing and transmitting information
    8. Telephone techniques
F. Medicolegal Guidelines & Requirements
    2. Legislation
H. Equipment
    1. Equipment operation

M. Resource Information and Community Services
    2. Appropriate referrals
P. Office Policies and Procedures
    3. Instructions for patients with special needs

RMA
II. Administrative Medical Assisting
    C. Medical Receptionist/Secretarial/Clerical
        4. Oral (and written) communication

CMAS
8. Medical Office Management
    • Office communications

COMPETENCY ASSESSMENT

Procedure 12-1 Answering and Screening Incoming Calls

Performance Objectives: To answer telephone calls professionally, acquiring all necessary information from the caller, documenting it correctly, and properly acting on it. Perform this objective within 15 minutes with a minimum score of 60 points.

Supplies/Equipment: Telephone, appointment calendar, message pad, pen or pencil, notepad, triage/assessment protocols

Charting/Documentation: Enter appropriate documentation/charting in the box.

_____

_____

_____

_____

Instructor's/Evaluator's Comments and Suggestions:

_____

_____

_____

_____

_____

_____

SKILLS CHECKLIST Procedure 12-1: Answering and Screening Incoming Calls

Name _____

Date _____

No.	Skill	Check #1 20 pts ea	Check #2 10 pts ea	Check #3 5 pts ea	Notes
1	Prepare materials.				
2	Answer phone within three rings.				
3	Answer with preferred greeting, speaking clearly.				
4	Ask for caller's name and determine if call is an emergency.				
5	Focus on the caller.				
6	Repeat the information back to the patient.				
7	Follow established office protocol for triaging.				
8	Keep a notepad handy to jot down the patient's name and number. Repeat information back to caller.				
9	Ask caller for any other questions.				
10	End call courteously.				
11	Let the caller hang up first.				
12	Document information and record future necessary actions.				
Student's Total Points					
Points Possible		240	120	60	
Final Score (Student's Total Points / Possible Points)					

	Notes
Start time:	
End time:	
Total time: (15 min goal)	

COMPETENCY ASSESSMENT

Procedure 12-2 Transferring a Call

Performance Objectives: To transfer a call directly to the individual who can handle the call in an efficient and professional manner. Perform this objective within 3 minutes with a minimum score of 40 points.

Supplies/Equipment: Telephone, message pad, black ink pen, notepad, interoffice telephone directory

Charting/Documentation: Enter appropriate documentation/charting in the box.

_____

_____

_____

_____

Instructor's/Evaluator's Comments and Suggestions:

_____

_____

_____

_____

_____

SKILLS CHECKLIST Procedure 12-2: Transferring a Call

Name _____

Date _____

No.	Skill	Check #1 20 pts ea	Check #2 10 pts ea	Check #3 5 pts ea	Notes
1	Answer the call as outlined in Procedure 12-1.				
2	Obtain the name and phone number of individual, and write down notes regarding situation.				
3	Determine best person to assist the caller.				
4	Ask caller for permission before placing him or her on hold.				
5	Return to caller and thank him or her for holding.				
6	Give name and extension of person you are transferring to.				
7	Follow your telephone system's procedure for transferring the call.				
8	Follow up to be sure the call transferred correctly.				
Student's Total Points					
Points Possible		160	80	40	
Final Score (Student's Total Points / Possible Points)					

	Notes
Start time:	
End time:	
Total time: (3 min goal)	

COMPETENCY ASSESSMENT
Procedure 12-3 Taking a Telephone Message

Performance Objectives: To record an accurate message and follow up as required. Perform this objective within 5 minutes with a minimum score of 55 points.

Supplies/Equipment: Telephone, message pad, black ink pen, notepad, clock or watch

Charting/Documentation: Enter appropriate documentation/charting in the box.

_____

_____

_____

_____

Instructor's/Evaluator's Comments and Suggestions:

_____

_____

_____

_____

_____

_____

SKILLS CHECKLIST Procedure 12-3: Taking a Telephone Message

Name _____

Date _____

No.	Skill	Check #1 20 pts ea	Check #2 10 pts ea	Check #3 5 pts ea	Notes
1	Answer the phone following the steps outlined in Procedure 12-1.				
2	Use a message pad to gather the required information.				
	a. Name of person calling and numbers				
	b. Date and time call was received				
	c. Who the call is for				
	d. Reason for the call				
	e. Action to be taken				
	f. Your name/initials				
3	Repeat the above information back to the caller.				
4	If the patient already has a medical record, attach the phone message to it.				
5	Maintain copies of all calls.				
Student's Total Points					
Points Possible		220	110	55	
Final Score (Student's Total Points / Possible Points)					

	Notes
Start time:	
End time:	
Total time: (5 min goal)	

COMPETENCY ASSESSMENT
Procedure 12-4 Handling Problem Calls

Performance Objectives: To handle calls in a positive and professional manner while providing necessary comfort, empathy, and information to the caller to resolve the problem. Perform this objective within 15 minutes with a minimum score of 65 points.

Supplies/Equipment: Telephone, message pad, pen or pencil

Charting/Documentation: Enter appropriate documentation/charting in the box.

_____

_____

_____

_____

Instructor's/Evaluator's Comments and Suggestions:

_____

_____

_____

_____

_____

_____

SKILLS CHECKLIST Procedure 12-4: Handling Problem Calls

Name _____

Date _____

No.	Skill	Check #1 20 pts ea	Check #2 10 pts ea	Check #3 5 pts ea	Notes
1	Answer the call as outlined in Procedure 12-1.				
2	Remain calm and avoid becoming upset.				
3	Lower your voice both in pitch and volume.				
4	Listen to what the caller is upset about, then paraphrase back to the caller for verification.				
5	Use the words "I understand."				
6	Do not take the call personally.				
7	Offer assistance.				
8	Document the call accurately.				
9	If caller is hysterical or frightened, speak in a soothing voice.				
10	If the call is an emergency, begin triage procedures as needed.				
11	Always have the caller repeat instructions.				
12	Finalize and follow through on action to be taken.				
13	Always report problem calls to the office manager.				
Student's Total Points					
Points Possible		260	130	65	
Final Score (Student's Total Points / Possible Points)					

	Notes
Start time:	
End time:	
Total time: (15 min goal)	

COMPETENCY ASSESSMENT

Procedure 12-5 Placing Outgoing Calls

Performance Objectives: To place calls efficiently and effectively. Perform this objective within 3 minutes with a minimum score of 25 points.

Supplies/Equipment: Telephone, notepad, pen or pencil, all materials specifically applicable to the call

Charting/Documentation: Enter appropriate documentation/charting in the box.

_____

_____

_____

_____

Instructor's/Evaluator's Comments and Suggestions:

_____

_____

_____

_____

_____

SKILLS CHECKLIST Procedure 12-5: Placing Outgoing Calls

Name _____

Date _____

No.	Skill	Check #1 20 pts ea	Check #2 10 pts ea	Check #3 5 pts ea	Notes
1	Preplan the call by preparing all materials.				
2	Make calls from a location that will not be disrupted.				
3	Schedule specific times of the day for calls. Be aware of time zones.				
4	Use appropriate language and tone, and follow proper telephone techniques.				
5	Document appropriately.				
Student's Total Points					
Points Possible		100	50	25	
Final Score (Student's Total Points / Possible Points)					

	Notes
Start time:	
End time:	
Total time: (3 min goal)	

COMPETENCY ASSESSMENT

Procedure 12-6 Recording a Telephone Message on an Answering Device or Voice Mail System

Performance Objectives: To provide clear and precise instructions to the caller when medical staff is not available to answer the call immediately. The words should be spoken clearly in a pleasant and well-modulated tone. Perform this objective within 15 minutes with a minimum score of 25 points.

Supplies/Equipment: Telephone and recording device, prepared written message to record

Charting/Documentation: Enter appropriate documentation/charting in the box.

_____

_____

_____

_____

Instructor's/Evaluator's Comments and Suggestions:

_____

_____

_____

_____

_____

_____

SKILLS CHECKLIST Procedure 12-6: Recording a Telephone Message on an Answering Device or Voice Mail System

Name _____

Date _____

No.	Skill	Check #1 20 pts ea	Check #2 10 pts ea	Check #3 5 pts ea	Notes
1	Write out message to be recorded.				
2	Check for completeness and accuracy, and read message aloud to determine its length.				
3	Record the message when distractions and noise are at a minimum.				
4	Play the message back to verify that it is accurate and includes all necessary information.				
5	Set the message device to the recorded message when you are not available to answer.				
Student's Total Points					
Points Possible		100	50	25	
Final Score (Student's Total Points / Possible Points)					

	Notes
Start time:	
End time:	
Total time: (15 min goal)	

EVALUATION OF CHAPTER KNOWLEDGE

Evaluate your own strengths and weaknesses in communicating with others on the telephone, performing triage, directing calls, and understanding telephone systems and technology.

Skills	Student Self-Evaluation		
	Good	Average	Poor
I can adhere to the principles of preserving patient confidentiality.	——	——	——
I project empathy and enthusiasm.	——	——	——
I understand telephone procedures for new and existing patient appointments.	——	——	——
I have the ability to triage and respond to medical emergencies.	——	——	——
I possess good listening skills.	——	——	——
I can receive, prioritize, organize, and transmit information.	——	——	——
I understand the principles of successful telephone communication.	——	——	——
I can perform effective telephone triage.	——	——	——
I understand the use of communication technology such as a fax machine, automated routing units, and e-mail.	——	——	——
I have the ability to communicate effectively with people at their levels of understanding.	——	——	——
I can demonstrate the ability to make outgoing calls.	——	——	——
I can serve as an effective liaison between the physician and others.	——	——	——
I can perform within ethical boundaries.	——	——	——
I practice within the scope of my training and expertise.	——	——	——

CHAPTER 13

Patient Scheduling

CHAPTER PRE-TEST

Perform this test without looking at the book. This is just to see how well you have understood and can recall the information in this chapter after you have read it, but before you have completed the workbook exercises. You will not be graded on this portion (other than the grade you give yourself). Justify any "false" answers.

1. Circle the letter that lists correct types of scheduling systems:
   a. wave, modified wave, double booking, a mile-a-minute
   b. open hours, wave, clustering, stream
   c. first-come first-served, open hours, clustering

2. Below are guidelines to scheduling. Which one is correct?
   a. Urgent calls should be sent to the hospital, where they are better equipped to handle them.
   b. Urgent calls should be triaged/assessed before determining the best course of action.
   c. Referrals by other physicians need to be seen immediately.
   d. Appointments for pharmaceutical and medical supply representatives should be referred to the physician.

3. Information that should be obtained from all new patients includes all but which one of the following?
   a. the patient's full legal name
   b. the patient's birth date
   c. the patient's address and telephone numbers
   d. the patient's symptoms
   e. the patient's insurance information
   f. the patient's family health history

4. All medical offices are changing to electronic appointment scheduling. (T or F)

5. When a patient misses an appointment, we:
   a. call them to reschedule
   b. let them contact us
   c. release them from our practice
   d. charge them for our time

INTRODUCTION

The effective scheduling of patient appointments is an essential skill of the medical assistant. Achieving efficient patient flow requires that the medical assistant coordinate the schedules of physicians, staff, and patients. Use of staff and physical facilities are also considered in selecting the proper scheduling system. When scheduling appointments, medical assistants draw on administrative and computer skills, as well as communication skills. By considering and respecting the needs, time, and comfort of the patient, the medical assistant creates a positive impression of the physician and the medical practice.

PERFORMANCE OBJECTIVES

After successful completion of this chapter you will be able to list and describe six major scheduling options, explaining the advantages and disadvantages of each; list some scheduling guidelines and state the rationales for them; explain the importance of triaging calls and how to handle certain situations you might encounter; be able to demonstrate the proper documentation processes for canceled and missed appointments; and be able to review the office protocols and procedures for patients checking in for appointments. You will be able to establish a schedule matrix given the parameters, and also be able to successfully schedule an outpatient procedure or surgery according to the needs of your patient and physician–employer. *The following statements are related to your learning objectives for this chapter. Fill in the blanks with the appropriate term(s).*

Six major options in scheduling include (1) _____, (2) _____, (3) _____, (4) _____, (5) _____, and (6) _____. One of the advantages of wave scheduling is that it can accommodate (7) _____ appointments. One of the staffing requirements when using wave scheduling is that the personnel must be skilled in (8) _____. Guidelines for scheduling appointments depend on many variables. Six of those variables are (9) _____, (10) _____, (11) _____, (12) _____, (13) _____, and (14) _____. When a patient misses an appointment, the medical assistant should contact the patient and attempt to (15) _____ the appointment. Both the missed appointment and the rescheduled appointment should be (16) _____ in the patient's medical record. When scheduling inpatient admissions and surgeries and outpatient procedures, it is important to consider the (17) _____ of the patient, the physician(s), and the facilities, as well as the equipment and personnel, depending on the services being scheduled.

VOCABULARY BUILDER

Find the words below that are misspelled; circle them, and then correctly spell them in the spaces provided. Then replace the highlighted words in the following paragraph with the correct vocabulary terms from the list. (Be sure to spell them all correctly!)

clustering
double booking
encription technology
estableshed patient
matrics

modified wave scheduling
new patient
no-show
open hours
practice based

slack time
stream scheduling
triage
wave scheduling

_____ _____ _____

1. _____ Inner City Health Care reserves 9 AM to 12 PM on Thursday mornings for walk-in patients who are seen on a first-come, first-served basis within that time frame.

2. _____ At the offices of Drs. Lewis and King, Ellen Armstrong, CMA, schedules Mary O'Keefe for a 1:00 PM appointment and Martin Gordon for a 1:00 PM appointment with Dr. Winston Lewis.

3. _____ Lenny Taylor, an older adult patient with mild dementia, forgets his third appointment with Dr. James Whitney.

4. _____ At Inner City Health Care, vaccinations are scheduled every 10 minutes from 10 AM to 12:20 PM on Mondays; Tuesday office hours are reserved for new patients only.

5. _____ Three patients are scheduled to receive treatments in the first half hour of every hour.

6. _____ Ellen Armstrong, CMA, takes a complete current medical history from patient Lourdes Austen on her first visit to Dr. Elizabeth King.

7. _____ Joe Guerrero, CMA, asks patient Martin Gordon if the personal information in his medical chart is complete and up to date before escorting him to the examination room to be seen by Dr. Winston Lewis.

8. _____ Dr. Elizabeth King prefers to see patients for regular gynecologic examinations in consecutive appointments from 8:30 AM to 11:30 AM and patients who are pregnant from 1:00 PM to 3:30 PM.

9. _____ When patient Herb Fowler calls to set up an appointment with Dr. Winston Lewis for his chronic cough, Ellen Armstrong, CMA, asks Herb a series of screening questions to ascertain the nature, extent, and urgency of his condition.

10. _____ Dr. Winston Lewis prefers that two or more patients be scheduled at 30 or 60 minute intervals on a continuous basis throughout the day.

11. _____ An ophthalmologist schedules three patients at the beginning of each hour for comprehensive examinations, followed by single appointments every 10 to 20 minutes during the rest of the hour for quick, follow-up procedures such as removing eye patches or instilling eyedrops.

12. _____ Ellen Armstrong, CMA, uses empty or unscheduled periods for dictation or processing paperwork.

13. _____ On the 15th day of each month, office manager Walter Seals, CMA, who is responsible for efficient patient flow at Inner City Health Care, asks each of the urgent care center's five physicians to confirm their scheduling commitments for the upcoming month to block off unavailable times in the appointment book.

14. _____ The medical assistant uses software to protect the patients' confidentiality in electronic format.

Appointment Book Matrix and Scheduling Activity

Student's Name: _____ Date: _____

Complete the appointment book in Figure 13-1 for Drs. Lewis and King according to the instructions in the appropriate Learning Review exercises.

		LEWIS & KING, MD 2501 CENTER STREET NORTHBOROUGH, OH 12345	
Friday, Feb. 7		**Dr. Lewis**	**Dr. King**
7	30		
	45		
8	00		
	15		
	30		
	45		
9	00		
	15		
	30		
	45		
10	00		
	15		
	30		
	45		

Figure 13-1

11	00		
	15		
	30		
	45		
12	00		
	15		
	30		
	45		
1	00		
	15		
	30		
	45		
2	00		
	15		
	30		
	45		
3	00		
	15		
	30		
	45		
4	00		

Figure 13-1 (continued)

LEARNING REVIEW

1. The first step in scheduling appointments is to establish an appointment matrix. The matrix blocks off time during the day that is used for purposes other than patient appointments and is unavailable for patient scheduling. Using the information below, complete the appointment book (see Figure 13-1) to establish an appointment matrix for the offices of Drs. Lewis and King on Friday, February 7. Physicians' commitments should be entered with a red pen.

    Dr. King's commitments: Aerobics 7:30–8:00 AM; hospital rounds 8:00–9:00 AM; 12:30–1:30 PM lunch for local chapter of American Medical Women's Association; 2:45–3:15 PM weekly meeting with office managers Marilyn Johnson and Shirley Brooks; 3:45–5:00 PM community lecture sponsored by Planned Parenthood.

    Dr. Lewis's commitments: 7:30–8:30 AM breakfast meeting with current president of the State Medical Society; 1:00–1:30 PM lunch in office; 3:30 PM golf with Dr. Wilson.

2. A. Appointment books are legal documents recording patient flow. For a manual appointment system, where pencil is used for ease in rescheduling, what can the medical assistant do to ensure that a permanent record is secured?

    _____

    _____

    _____

    _____

    For a computerized appointment system, what can a medical assistant do to ensure that a permanent record of patient flow is secured?

    _____

    _____

    B. Name two primary goals in determining the best method for scheduling patient appointments:

    (1) _____

    _____

    (2) _____

    _____

    C. What is the typical scheduling time for each of the following types of office visits for an internal medicine practice?

    (1) Patient consultation _____

    (2) Established patient routine follow-up _____

    (3) New patient _____

    (4) Complete physical examination _____

    (5) Cold/flu symptoms _____

    (6) Vaccination _____

D. Using the appointment book (Figure 13-2), schedule the following appointments for Drs. Lewis and King for Friday, February 7.

Dr. King   Lourdes Austen; 651-8282; HMO insurance; complete physical examination and consultation regarding pregnancy after breast cancer; 1 hour, check-up and laboratory work.

Margaret Thomas; 651-0020; PPO insurance; chief complaint: Parkinson's disease; routine follow-up and vitamin B_{12} injection; 45 minutes.

Abigail Johnson; 389-2631; chief complaint: hypertension, diabetes mellitus, and angina; routine follow-up examination, 30 minutes.

Susan Marshall; 628-9981; PPO insurance; chief complaint: intense emotional stress, heart palpitations; complete examination and ECG; 1 hour.

Herb Fowler; 639-1134; chief complaint: ankle sprain from recent fall in garage; recheck, 15 minutes.

Dr. Lewis   Charles Williams; 689-1144; Blue Cross/Blue Shield; chief complaint: recurrent chest pain; physical examination and administer Holter monitor; 1 hour.

Rowena Lawrence; 628-3485; HMO insurance; chief complaint: hoarseness and bloody sputum; physical examination and laboratory work, 1 hour.

Mark Johnson; 635-1111; HMO insurance; chief complaint: chronic lower back pain; recheck, 15 minutes.

Helen Armstrong; 628-9967; PPO insurance; new patient, self-referred; chief complaint: mild edema in right leg; physical examination, 1 hour.

Larry Melnick; 635-7721; accountant; 1 hour to discuss income statement for previous year and preparation of tax returns for the medical practice.

Marsha Lewis; 628-9986; representative of pharmaceutical company; sales meeting; 15 minutes.

Martin Gordon; 635-9834; HMO insurance; chief complaint: prostate cancer; routine follow-up; 30 minutes.

Veronica Hallett; 635-4432; PPO insurance; chief complaint: persistent dermatitis; follow-up, 15 minutes.

Anne Ortiz; 628-5467; new patient, referred by Dr. John Elmos; Blue Cross/Blue Shield; chief complaint: recurring stomach problems; 45 minutes.

3. Daily appointment sheets provide permanent records for legal risk management and are excellent tools for quality management of patient flow. Appointment sheets can be used to check off patients seen, no-shows, and cancellations. A pocket-sized edition of the daily appointment sheet is often given to the physician for easy referral. Compile a daily patient appointment sheet for Dr. Winston Lewis based on your scheduling of his appointments into the appointment matrix at the beginning of the Learning Review (see Question 1).

Daily Appointment Sheet   Dr. Lewis   Friday, February 7

Appointment Time	Patient Name	Time Allotted	Reason for Visit

Figure 13-2

4. Daily worksheets include not only patient appointments, but all other physician and staff appointments as well. Daily worksheets are helpful tools that indicate blocks of time in any given day that are booked for any purpose and thus are not available as scheduling time to see patients. Compile a daily worksheet (Figure 13-3) based on Dr. Elizabeth King's schedule for Friday, February 7.

Daily Workheet   Dr. King   Friday, February 7

Time	Appointment	Expected Length of Appointment	Reason for Appointment

Figure 13-3

5. A. What are six variables involved in the process of scheduling appointments for patients and other visitors to the ambulatory care setting?

   (1) _____

   (2) _____

   (3) _____

   (4) _____

   (5) _____

   (6) _____

   B. Patient Flow Analysis sheets help medical practices determine the effectiveness of patient scheduling and devise plans for improving a smooth patient flow through the ambulatory care setting. What kinds of issues can a study of these data reveal?

   _____

   _____

   _____

   _____

   _____

6. What are the five steps of scheduling a specific appointment time for a patient?

   (1) _____

   (2) _____

   (3) _____

   (4) _____

   (5) _____

7. Cancellations, emergencies, no-shows, and appointment changes can affect the appointment scheduling for any given day in the ambulatory care setting. Consider the appointment schedule for Drs. Lewis and King that you completed at the beginning of the Learning Review. Make the following adjustments.

   A. Mary O'Keefe calls at 8:45 AM when her 3-year-old son Chris woke with severe ear pain. The child is pulling on his right ear and has screamed uncontrollably for 45 minutes. Chris and Mary are established patients of Dr. King.

   This telephone call is triaged as an emergency requiring immediate attention. Reschedule appointments as necessary to give the patient an emergency 9:00 AM appointment with Dr. King; about a half hour should be reserved for the emergency. Describe your logic in determining how Dr. King's appointment schedule will be adjusted to handle the emergency situation.

   _____

   _____

   _____

   _____

   _____

B. Patient Mark Johnson is a no-show on Dr. Lewis's schedule. Mark the no-show appropriately on the appointment schedule. What other action must be taken to document Mr. Johnson's no-show status? Why is it important to accurately and completely document patient no-shows and cancellations?

_____

_____

_____

_____

C. Patient Martin Gordon calls to cancel his appointment with Dr. Lewis. He has rescheduled his appointment two weeks later at the same time.

(1) Mark the cancellation appropriately on the appointment schedule.

(2) (a) After documenting the appointment change in the patient chart, the medical assistant completes an appointment card (Figure 13-4) and mails it to Mr. Gordon as a reminder of his new appointment time.

LEWIS & KING, MD
2501 CENTER STREET
NORTHBOROUGH, OH 12345

M _____

has an appointment on

Mon. _____ at _____

Tues. _____ at _____

Wed. _____ at _____

Thurs. _____ at _____

Fri. _____ at _____

If unable to keep appointment, kindly give 24 hours notice.

Figure 13-4

(b) Two ways of reminding patients of upcoming appointments are to give the appointment card personally to the patient and to mail the card to the patient. Identify a third reminder system. What procedures must be observed to protect patient confidentiality when using this third method?

_____

_____

_____

_____

8. The best scheduling system for a practice is the one that effects good patient flow and proper use of staff and physical facilities.

   A. Identify seven scheduling styles.

   (1) _____

   (2) _____

   (3) _____

   (4) _____

   (5) _____

   (6) _____

   (7) _____

   B. For each medical practice or facility below, identify the best scheduling system and explain the reasoning behind your choice.

   (1) Hospital emergency room: _____

   _____

   _____

   (2) Laboratory for blood testing: _____

   _____

   _____

   (3) Two-physician group practice: _____

   _____

   _____

   (4) Urgent care center with emergency and clinic facilities: _____

   _____

   _____

9. Scheduling outpatient procedures:

   a. is done at the end of each day

   b. is best done with the patient present

   c. will be easier with a calendar visualized

   d. b and c

10. One principal above all else in scheduling for the office is:

   a. flexibility

   b. neatness

   c. accountability

   d. estimation

11. The type of scheduling that requires visits to be set up around patients with specific chronic aliments such as diabetes and hypertension is called:

    a. triaging

    b. referral appointments

    c. group appointments

    d. stream appointments

12. The general rule for no-shows and cancellations is that after _____ consecutive missed appointments, the physician will review the patient's record and could terminate care.

    a. five

    b. three

    c. two

    d. ten

13. What, more than anything else, determines the success of a day in the ambulatory care setting?

    a. patient care

    b. efficient patient flow

    c. operational functions

    d. interpersonal skills

CERTIFICATION REVIEW

These questions are designed to mimic the certification examinations. You can use these questions like a small "Certification Examination Study Guide," but this is not meant to take the place of the more extensive study guides. Use this portion to determine in what areas to concentrate your efforts when studying for the certification examination.

1. In scheduling, double booking means to keep two appointment books going for the same doctor. (T or F)

2. One major purpose of triage when scheduling appointments is to determine if the patient has an emergency or urgent situation/illness. (T or F)

3. After a patient has missed three appointments, most clinics refuse to schedule that patient again. (T or F)

4. The appointment book/record may be subpoenaed, and therefore is considered a legal document. (T or F)

5. Providing patients with appointment cards is an effective way to prevent missed appointments. (T or F)

CASE STUDY

When patient Lenore McDonell falls from the examination table and lacerates her arm while attempting an independent transfer from the table to her wheelchair, clinical medical assistant Joe Guerrero alerts Dr. Winston Lewis, and the two begin to implement emergency procedures to control Lenore's bleeding and assess damage to the arm. Lenore's fall occurred at the end of her appointment, a routine checkup with Dr. Lewis.

Administrative medical assistant Ellen Armstrong must adjust Dr. Lewis's schedule to accommodate the emergency situation. Martin Gordon, a man in his mid-60s diagnosed with prostate cancer, waits in the reception area for Dr. Lewis's next appointment. Mr. Gordon's appointment, a 6-month follow-up, is expected to take 30 minutes. Mr. Gordon is also being treated for depression related to his cancer diagnosis. Hope Smith, a new patient in good general health, is scheduled for a complete examination; she is due to arrive at the offices of Drs. Lewis and King at the Northborough Family Medical Group within 20 minutes. Jim Marshall, an impatient and aggressive businessman, is scheduled for the first afternoon appointment after Dr. Lewis's lunch commitment. Mr. Marshall's appointment, for a physical examination and ECG to investigate chest pains he has experienced recently, is expected to take 45 minutes. Dr. Lewis's schedule is completely booked for the rest of the day.

Discuss the following:
1. What scheduling alternatives will Ellen offer Mr. Gordon, who is already waiting in the reception area? What special considerations regarding Mr. Gordon should Ellen take into account and why?
2. What is Ellen's first action regarding Ms. Smith, Dr. Lewis's next patient due to arrive? What scheduling alternatives should Ellen offer to her?
3. What scheduling alternatives, if any, should Ellen present to Mr. Marshall? Explain your logic.
4. How is patient triage important to Ellen's rescheduling of Dr. Lewis's patients? What important administrative and communication skills will Ellen use to handle this emergency situation efficiently and professionally?

SELF-ASSESSMENT

1. When you call a doctor's office, do any of the following aggravate you? Do you think other people are aggravated by these?

   a. Being put on hold right away or too often

   b. The receptionist asking too many questions

   c. Not enough appointment time choices; that is, you have to wait too long for an appointment

   d. Not getting a real person; that is, having to listen to electronic choices and make selections

   e. Other (add your own idea) _____

   _____

2. Now go to each of the situations in Question 1 and determine an action that could alleviate all or some of the aggravation. Keep in mind that the situation might still exist (e.g., the receptionist might still have to ask a lot of questions), but how might he or she make the experience more pleasant?

3. When you visit a doctor's office, do any of the following aggravate you?

   a. The receptionist does not acknowledge you right away

   b. The wait is too long

   c. The waiting room is noisy, messy, or uncomfortable

   d. There are no magazines of interest to you

   e. Other (add your own idea) _____

   _____

4. Similar to the instructions in Question 2, go to each of the situations in Question 3 and determine solutions that could alleviate all or some of the causes of aggravation. Keep in mind that the solutions in this case are obvious and doable.

5. Think of your most pleasant interaction with a doctor's office as a patient making an appointment, scheduling a procedure, changing an appointment, or even canceling an appointment. What made the experience more pleasant? Was it the receptionist's voice? Tone? Actual words? The overall options? Or something else?

   As you enter your career as a medical assistant, try to remember how the patient feels. Try to recall situations that bother you when you are a patient. Try to keep these issues in mind and see if you can eliminate or alleviate them to make your patients as comfortable as possible. Maybe you are just the person who will help to make the experience of seeing a doctor more pleasant for your patients. Try to be like the person you thought of for Question 5. This is not an easy thing to do when you are busy and stressed. Can you think of ways you can remind yourself every day of these lessons?

CHAPTER POST-TEST

This is similar to the Pre-Test. Perform this test without looking at the book. This is just to see how well you have understood and can recall the information presented in this chapter after you have studied it and completed the workbook exercises. You will not be graded on this portion (other than the grade you give yourself), but this is an excellent preparation for your instructor's test. You may use this Post-Test to determine what areas you need to study more. Justify any "false" answers.

1. Circle the letter that lists correct types of scheduling systems:

   a. modified wave, wave, clustering, and mile-a-minute

   b. stream, open hours, wave, grouping, separating

   c. first-come first-served, open hours, clustering

   d. open hours, wave, clustering, stream

2. Below are guidelines to scheduling. Which one is correct?

  a. Urgent calls should be scheduled into the next available appointment time.

  b. Urgent calls should be sent to the hospital, where they are better equipped to handle them.

  c. Calls from other physicians should be put through to the physician immediately, if possible.

  d. Appointments for pharmaceutical and medical supply representatives should be referred to the physician.

3. Information that should be obtained from all new patients includes all but which one of the following?

  a. the patient's full legal name

  b. the patient's birth date

  c. the patient's address and telephone numbers

  d. the patient's place of employment

  e. the patient's symptoms

  f. the patient's insurance information

4. Many medical offices are changing to electronic appointment scheduling. (T or F)

5. When a patient misses an appointment, we document it, and then we:

  a. call them to reschedule

  b. let them contact us

  c. release them from our practice

  d. charge them for our time

CERTIFICATION CRITERIA CHECKLIST

As you go through your education and training, keep in mind the national certification examination that you will take when you graduate. Each chapter of the textbook and workbook covers a different section of the examination criteria. To keep track of your preparation for the certification examination, turn to the back of this workbook and highlight the following CMA, RMA, or CMAS certification examination criteria (if you have already highlighted them from a previous chapter, put a check mark by the criteria):

CMA
E. Communication
     8. Telephone techniques
H. Equipment
     1. Equipment operation
I. Computer Concepts
     3. Computer applications
L. Scheduling and Monitoring Appointments

N.   Managing Physician's Professional Schedule and Travel
     3.   Integrating meetings and travel with office schedule

RMA

II.   Administrative Medical Assisting
     C.   Medical Receptionist/Secretarial/Clerical
          2.   Reception
          3.   Scheduling

CMAS

3.   Medical Office Clerical Assisting
     •   Appointment management and scheduling

COMPETENCY ASSESSMENT
Procedure 13-1 Checking In Patients

Performance Objectives: To ensure the patient is given prompt and proper care; to meet legal safeguards for documentation. Perform this objective within 25 minutes with a minimum score of 35 points.

Supplies/Equipment: Patient chart, black ink pen, required forms, check-in list or appointment book

Charting/Documentation: Enter appropriate documentation/charting in the box.

_____

_____

_____

_____

Instructor's/Evaluator's Comments and Suggestions:

_____

_____

_____

_____

_____

_____

SKILLS CHECKLIST Procedure 13-1: Checking In Patients

Name _____

Date _____

No.	Skill	Check #1 20 pts ea	Check #2 10 pts ea	Check #3 5 pts ea	Notes
1	Prepare a list of patients to be seen and assemble the charts.				
2	Check charts to see that everything is up to date.				
3	Acknowledge patients when they arrive.				
4	Check patient in, review vital information, and protect patient's privacy.				
5	Indicate patients arrival on daily worksheet and computer system.				
6	Ask patient to be seated and indicate wait time.				
7	Following office policy, place the chart where it can be picked up to route the patient to the appropriate location for the visit.				
	Student's Total Points				
	Points Possible	140	70	35	
	Final Score (Student's Total Points / Possible Points)				

	Notes
Start time:	
End time:	
Total time: (25 min goal)	

COMPETENCY ASSESSMENT

Procedure 13-2 Cancellation Procedures

Performance Objectives: To protect the physician from legal complications; to free up care time for other patients; and to assure quality patient care. Perform this objective within 15 minutes with a minimum score of 20 points.

Supplies/Equipment: Patient chart, red ink pen, check-in list or appointment book

Charting/Documentation: Enter appropriate documentation/charting in the box.

_____

_____

_____

_____

Instructor's/Evaluator's Comments and Suggestions:

_____

_____

_____

_____

_____

_____

SKILLS CHECKLIST Procedure 13-2: Cancellation Procedures

Name _____

Date _____

No.	Skill	Check #1 20 pts ea	Check #2 10 pts ea	Check #3 5 pts ea	Notes
1	Indicate on the appointment sheet all appointments that were changed, canceled, or did not show.				
2	Reschedule those appointments by calling the patients.				
3	If unable to reschedule, record a reminder in the tickler file.				
4	Document action taken in the patient's medical record/ chart.				
Student's Total Points					
Points Possible		80	40	20	
Final Score (Student's Total Points / Possible Points)					

	Notes
Start time:	
End time:	
Total time: (15 min goal)	

COMPETENCY ASSESSMENT
Procedure 13-3 Establishing the Appointment Matrix

Performance Objectives: To have a current and accurate record of appointment times available for scheduling patient visits. Perform this objective within 25 minutes with a minimum score of 25 points.

Supplies/Equipment: Appointment scheduler, physician's schedule, staff schedule, office calendar

Charting/Documentation: Enter appropriate documentation/charting in the box.

_____

_____

_____

_____

Instructor's/Evaluator's Comments and Suggestions:

_____

_____

_____

_____

_____

SKILLS CHECKLIST Procedure 13-3: Establishing the Appointment Matrix

Name _____

Date _____

No.	Skill	Check #1 20 pts ea	Check #2 10 pts ea	Check #3 5 pts ea	Notes
1	Mark in appointment book times that are not to be scheduled.				
2	Indicate all vacations, holidays, and other office closures.				
3	Note all physician meetings, hospital rounds, appointments, conferences, vacations, and other prescheduled commitments.				
4	Highlight the time frame for specific procedures.				
5	Have clearly established guidelines for scheduling specific types of appointments and procedures.				
	Student's Total Points				
	Points Possible	100	50	25	
	Final Score (Student's Total Points / Possible Points)				

	Notes
Start time:	
End time:	
Total time: (25 min goal)	

COMPETENCY ASSESSMENT

Procedure 13-4 Scheduling of Inpatient and Outpatient Admissions and Procedures

Performance Objectives: To assist patients in scheduling inpatient and outpatient admissions and procedures ordered by the physician. Perform this objective within 20 minutes with a minimum score of 45 points.

Supplies/Equipment: Calendar, black ink pen, telephone, referral slip, patient's schedule/calendar, physician's requests/orders regarding procedure/admittance

Charting/Documentation: Enter appropriate documentation/charting in the box.

_____

_____

_____

_____

Instructor's/Evaluator's Comments and Suggestions:

_____

_____

_____

_____

_____

_____

SKILLS CHECKLIST Procedure 13-4: Scheduling of Inpatient and Outpatient Admissions and Procedures

Name _____

Date _____

No.	Skill	Check #1 20 pts ea	Check #2 10 pts ea	Check #3 5 pts ea	Notes
1	Ensure privacy. Clarify with the patients that they understand the inpatient admission or outpatient procedure ordered.				
2	If required, seek permission from the patient's insurance company for the procedure or admissions.				
3	Produce a large, easily read calendar and check to see if the patient has one.				
4	Place telephone call to the facility. Identify yourself, your physician, your clinic, and the reason for calling.				
5	Identify any urgency. Request next available appointment.				
6	Confer with the patient for an immediate response.				
7	Provide receiver pertinent information related to the patient.				
8	Request special instructions or advanced data.				
9	Complete the referral slip for the patient; send or fax a copy to referred facility.				
Student's Total Points					
Points Possible		180	90	45	
Final Score (Student's Total Points / Possible Points)					

	Notes
Start time:	
End time:	
Total time: (20 min goal)	

COMPETENCY ASSESSMENT

Procedure 13-5 Making an Appointment on the Telephone

Performance Objectives: To schedule an appointment entering information in the appointment schedule according to office policy. Perform this objective within 15 minutes with a minimum score of 40 points.

Supplies/Equipment: Telephone, black ink pen, calendar, appointment book/computer screen/appointment worksheet

Charting/Documentation: Enter appropriate documentation/charting in the box.

_____

_____

_____

_____

Instructor's/Evaluator's Comments and Suggestions:

_____

_____

_____

_____

_____

_____

SKILLS CHECKLIST Procedure 13-5: Making an Appointment on the Telephone

Name _____

Date _____

No.	Skill	Check #1 20 pts ea	Check #2 10 pts ea	Check #3 5 pts ea	Notes
1	Answer the call following the steps outlined in Procedure 12-1.				
2	Make notes on your personal log sheet of patient's name and reason for calling.				
3	Determine if patient is new or established, physician to be seen, and reason for appointment.				
4	Discuss with the patient any special scheduling needs and search for an available time.				
5	Enter patient's name into the schedule.				
6	Repeat the date and time, and provide necessary instructions.				
7	End the call politely.				
8	Make certain all necessary information was transferred from your telephone log to appointment schedule. Draw line through your notes.				
Student's Total Points					
Points Possible		160	80	40	
Final Score (Student's Total Points / Possible Points)					

	Notes
Start time:	
End time:	
Total time: (15 min goal)	

EVALUATION OF CHAPTER KNOWLEDGE

Skills	Student Self-Evaluation		
	Good	Average	Poor
I can choose appropriate scheduling tools and can describe advantages of each.	_____	_____	_____
I am able to establish an appointment matrix.	_____	_____	_____
I can prepare the daily appointment sheet.	_____	_____	_____
I can prepare the daily worksheet.	_____	_____	_____
I understand the importance of triage in scheduling patient appointments.	_____	_____	_____
I understand basic considerations in scheduling appointments.	_____	_____	_____
I know how to review procedures for cancellations, no-shows, and appointment changes.	_____	_____	_____
I know how to review procedures for patients checking in.	_____	_____	_____
I can recall three types of reminder systems.	_____	_____	_____
I can review six major scheduling systems.	_____	_____	_____
I recognize the importance of communication skills in the scheduling process.	_____	_____	_____

CHAPTER 14

Medical Records Management

CHAPTER PRE-TEST

Perform this test without looking at the book. This is just to see how well you have understood and can recall the information in this chapter after you have read it, but before you have completed the workbook exercises. You will not be graded on this portion (other than the grade you give yourself). Justify any "false" answers.

1. Out guides indicate when patient charts are out of order. (T or F)

2. Which of the following is not an important skill to have when filing?
   a. You should know the alphabet.
   b. You should know the basic rules of filing.
   c. You should pay attention to details.
   d. You should be good at math.

3. Medical records are important for many reasons. They provide information for medical care, legal protection, and research purposes. (T or F)

4. It is acceptable to release medical information to family members as long as they can show proper picture identification. (T or F)

5. When charting, you should write every detail of your conversation with the patient. (T or F)

6. All medical filing systems are based on the alphabet. (T or F)

INTRODUCTION

Accurate filing of patient medical records is an essential administrative task in the ambulatory care setting. To provide the highest quality care, patient medical records and other important files must be easily and promptly accessed by the physician and other members of the health care team.

The contents of all medical charts and other files must be kept complete and up to date. Medical assisting students can use this workbook chapter to review the filing systems commonly used in the ambulatory care setting and the correct procedures for medical records management.

PERFORMANCE OBJECTIVES

After successful completion of this chapter you should be able to explain the importance of medical records; discuss several methods of filing medical records, the rules for filing, and the order and steps for filing medical documents into the patient's chart or medical record, and describe several variations of filing systems. You should be able to define words such as tickler files, release marks, checkout systems, and cross-referencing. You should have a basic understanding of computer applications for medical records. You should know how an electronic medical record differs from a paper system in regard to retrieval, storage, making changes/corrections, access/transfers, and confidentiality. *The following statements are related to your learning objectives. Fill in the blanks with the appropriate term(s).*

There are five main purposes for medical records in the ambulatory care setting. One is to provide a base for (1) _____ patient care. Another is to provide (2) _____ and (3) _____ communications as necessary. A third purpose is to (4) _____ a pattern to signal the physician of patient needs. The fourth purpose is to serve as a (5) _____ for legal information necessary to (6) _____ physicians, (7) _____, and patients. The fifth and final purpose is to provide clinical data for (8) _____. When filing documents into a medical record/chart, there are certain procedural steps that should be followed for efficiency. The steps are (9) _____, (10) _____, (11) _____, and finally, (12) _____. There are many different methods of filing; some are alphabetical, some are numeric, and some are filed according to (13) _____. A (14) _____ _____ is a card system that helps you remember when an action is necessary in the future. Having the doctor initial laboratory reports before they are filed is a good example of (15) _____ _____ and helps to ensure the reports are not filed until the doctor has seen them. (16) _____ consist of "place holders" sometimes called "out sheets," or (17) _____. Medical records that are kept on computer are called (18) _____ and have distinct advantages and disadvantages. Regardless of how records are kept, patient (19) _____ is always a major concern, and safeguards must be in place to prevent unauthorized persons from seeing private medical information.

VOCABULARY BUILDER

Fill in the blanks in the following sentences using the words listed below.

accession record
captions
coding
consecutive or serial filing
cross-reference
indexing

key unit
nonconsecutive filing
out guide
problem-oriented medical
    record (POMR)
purging

shingling
SOAP
source-oriented medical
    record (SOMR)
tickler file
units

1. To remember to check with the reference laboratory on Friday to obtain patient Martin Gordon's test results, Ellen Armstrong, CMA places a note in her _____.

2. When using the _____ approach for all progress notes, Dr. Lewis enters information about a patient's problem in this order: S—subjective impressions; O—objective clinical evidence; A—assessment or diagnosis; P—plans for further studies, treatment, or management.

3. Every 6 months, Marilyn Johnson, CMA, follows office policy and procedures for _____ _____ inactive files to remove and archive those not in active use.

4. The organized method of identifying and separating items to be filed into small subunits is accomplished with the use of _____ units.

5. When Liz Corbin, CMA, retrieves Annette Samuels's chart for Dr. Woo, she places an _____ in the filing cabinet to show that the file has been removed from storage.

6. When returning a patient's chart to the filing cabinet, Walter Seals, CMA, inspects the patient's name to identify the indexing _____.

7. The _____ is a journal (or computer listing) where numbers in a numeric filing system are preassigned. The log sequentially lists numbers to be used to assign to numeric records.

8. The _____ filing system uses groups of two, three, or four or more digits, such as the patient's social security number or telephone number, as the filing reference in a numeric filing system.

9. The file for Kent Memorial Hospital contains three indexing _____ to be considered when preparing the filing label.

10. If a _____ card is required in the alphabetic card file of a numeric filing system, such as when making note of an established patient's married name, a card is prepared that includes an X next to the file number to indicate that this card does not designate the primary location card for the file.

11. In the _____ system of recordkeeping, patient problems are identified by a number that corresponds to the charting relevant to that problem number; that is, asthma #1; dermatitis #2; and so on.

12. When a filing system other than alphabetic is being used, the proper _____ must be determined for the chart or file so it can be retrieved.

13. Ellen Armstrong, CMA, uses the _____ method for filing laboratory reports; the reports are stacked across the page with the most recent report placed on top of the previous one.

14. Ellen Armstrong, CMA, uses the _____ method for handling invoices, sales orders, and requisitions; each record is numbered and filed in ascending order.

15. _____ are used to identify major sections of file folders by more manageable subunits, such as GA-GE, or Miscellaneous. Captions are marked on the tabs of the guides.

16. Inner City Health Care uses the _____ method of recordkeeping, which groups information according to its origin; for example, laboratories, examinations, physician notes, consulting physicians, and other types of information.

LEARNING REVIEW

1. Assign the correct units to the following items to be filed using the rule for filing patient records that is listed for each.

   A. Names that are hyphenated are considered one unit.

      1. Jackson Hugh Levine-Dwyer

         unit 1_____ unit 2_____ unit 3_____

      2. Leslie Jane Poole-Petit

         unit 1_____ unit 2_____ unit 3_____

   B. Seniority units are indexed as the last indexing unit.

      1. Keith Wildasin Sr.

         unit 1_____ unit 2_____ unit 3_____

      2. Gerald Maggart III

         unit 1_____ unit 2_____ unit 3_____

   C. Titles are considered as separate indexing units. If the title appears with first and last names, the title is considered the last indexing unit.

      1. Dr. Louise Udolf

         unit 1_____ unit 2_____ unit 3_____

      2. Prof. Valerie Rajah

         unit 1_____ unit 2_____ unit 3_____

D. The names of individuals are assigned indexing units respectively: last name, first name, middle, and succeeding names.

1. Lindsay Adair Martin

unit 1_____ unit 2_____ unit 3_____

2. Abigail Sue Johnson

unit 1_____ unit 2_____ unit 3_____

E. When indexing names of married women, the name is indexed by the legal name.

1. Mary Jane O'Keefe (Mrs. John)

unit 1_____ unit 2_____ unit 3_____ unit 4_____

2. Nora Patrice Fowler (Mrs. Herb)

unit 1_____ unit 2_____ unit 3_____ unit 4_____

F. Foreign language units are indexed as one unit with the unit that follows. Spacing, punctuation, and capitalization are ignored.

1. Joseph Jack de la Hoya

unit 1_____ unit 2_____ unit 3_____

2. Maurice John van de Veer

unit 1_____ unit 2_____ unit 3_____

2. Using the numbers 1, 2, and 3, label the patient names in each group according to the correct filing order of names in an alphabetic filing system.

A. _____ Larry Peter Sanders

_____ Larry Paul Samuels

_____ Lawrence Paul Sanders

B. _____ James Edward Reed Sr.

_____ James Edward Reed

_____ James Edward Reed Jr.

C. _____ Lynn Elaine Brenner

_____ Lynn Ellen Brenner

_____ Lynn Eloise Brenner

D. _____ Patrick Sam Saint

_____ Patrick Sam St. Bartz

_____ Paul Sam Saint

3. Circle the right answer(s) from the choices below.

A. Jane O'Hara, CMA, is filing patient records using a nonconsecutive numeric filing system. For the patient file labeled 618 32 6445, what is unit 1?

1. 6445

2. 618

3. 32 6445

B. The most important reason for using numeric filing is that:

   1. it preserves patient confidentiality.

   2. a larger number of records can be easily filed.

   3. a computer can more readily read numeric filing labels.

C. Walter Seals, CMA, is filing using a consecutive numeric filing system. For the patient file labeled 67 843, what is unit 1?

   1. 3

   2. 6

   3. 843

D. Outgoing correspondence is:

   1. friendly correspondence

   2. correspondence sent out of the medical office

   3. correspondence to be thrown away

E. Karen Ritter, CMA, is filing patient files using a numeric filing system. She comes across a file for a patient who has not yet been assigned a number. Karen should:

   1. put the file in the miscellaneous numeric file section.

   2. put the file in a pending filing bin until the physician can assign a number.

   3. put the file directly behind the rest of the files.

F. An out guide should contain:

   1. a record of when the chart was removed and the name of the person who has the chart.

   2. the signature of the patient's physician

   3. a record of when the file is expected to be returned

4. State statutes have ruled that medical records are the property of the:

   a. state medical society

   b. ones who create them

   c. patient only

   d. none of the above

5. Any information to be released from the medical record:

   a. goes to medical insurance

   b. requires a physician's signature

   c. requires patient notification and approval

   d. requires a subpoena

6. Filing equipment:

   a. should have a locking capability

   b. is available in vertical or lateral styles

   c. is to be stored in an area accessible only to authorized personnel

   d. all of the above

7. EMR stands for:

    a. emergency room

    b. a popular color-coding system's trade name

    c. electronic medical records

    d. emergency medical rules

8. Release marks include:

    a. date stamp and initials

    b. out guides

    c. tabs

    d. SOAP

CERTIFICATION REVIEW

These questions are designed to mimic the certification examinations. You can use these questions like a small "Certification Examination Study Guide," but this is not meant to take the place of the more extensive study guides. Use this portion to determine in what areas to concentrate your efforts when studying for the certification examination.

1. The POMR is also known as:

    a. source-oriented medical record

    b. SOAP system

    c. traditional method

    d. problem-oriented medical record

    e. none of the above

2. SOAP stands for:

    a. a way to sanitize instruments

    b. patient electronic records

    c. a type of filing system

    d. a charting system

    e. none of the above

3. If a patient needs to return for another examination in 6 months, you might use a reminder system. What is the name of that system?

    a. reminder system

    b. recall system

    c. phone log

    d. tickler system

    e. out guide

4. The most common method of filing in today's medical office is:

    a. alphabetically

    b. numerically

    c. by insurance

    d. by subject

    e. color coding

5. If a medical document is filed in multiple places, you might use a(n):

    a. index

    b. out guide

    c. cross-reference

    d. multiple reference

    e. cross-filed card

CASE STUDY

At the offices of Drs. Lewis and King, co-office managers Marilyn Johnson and Shirley Brooks stress the importance of maintaining accurate, up-to-date, and complete documentation in all patient medical records. The practice uses the POMR method of recordkeeping for patient files within an alphabetical color-coded filing system. Drs. Lewis and King use the SOAP approach in charting patient progress notes. Twice each year, the office managers hold a special staff meeting devoted solely to a discussion of the filing system. The meeting is used to answer staff questions and consider ideas for streamlining the filing system to increase efficiency and ease of use.

Discuss the following:
1. Why is accurate, up-to-date, and complete documentation in patient medical records essential in the ambulatory care setting?
2. Why is the POMR system commonly used by family practice offices?
3. Why is a color-coding system effective in the ambulatory care setting?
4. How important is an effective, easy-to-use, and easy-to-access filing system to the efficiency of the ambulatory care setting?

SELF-ASSESSMENT

To perform this self-assessment, you must first perform an exercise: Go to your spice drawer, a stack of magazines, a bunch of bills/statements, or even your clothes closet, drawers, or the shelves you keep your towels on. Maybe organize something in your medical assisting classroom or laboratory area. Think of the best way to organize them. Is it by size, color, or both? Alphabetically? By date? Frequency of use? Perform the organization. What was the most difficult part; planning how to best accomplish it, or actually doing it? Did you have to take everything out and place it back in order, or were you able to just move things around? Was this a time-consuming exercise? Is the order now a useful tool? Did you have any decisions to make, such as do you file red pepper under red or pepper? Should your pants be organized with their matching tops, or should all the pants be together and all the tops together? Should the medications be organized in alphabetical order, or by classification (type of action)? Now choose another item to organize in a different way. How did this second exercise differ? I suspect your towels were organized by size or by color, whereas your spices would be organized alphabetically. Do you think another person would have chosen a different method? Who do you think decides in an office how a particular area is to be organized? Do you think there might be different ways? Let us pretend that your doctor's office has its patients' charts filed alphabetically, but now they are moving to more computerized records and want to change their files to a numeric system. Make a list of the supplies the staff will need, calculate the time it might take, and make up a plan on how to accomplish this (remember the files are still being used everyday). Does this seem like a major undertaking? Could any files be purged (pulled out of circulation) during this reorganization?

CHAPTER POST-TEST

This is similar to the Pre-Test. Perform this test without looking at the book. This is just to see how well you have understood and can recall the information presented in this chapter after you have studied it and completed the workbook exercises. You will not be graded on this portion (other than the grade you give yourself), but this is an excellent preparation for your instructor's test. You may use this Post-Test to determine what areas you need to study more. Justify any "false" answers.

1. When patient charts are out of order, we use out guides to help us see the error better. (T or F)

2. When filing, you need to be skilled in all but which one of the following?
   a. knowing the alphabet
   b. knowing the basic rules of filing
   c. being able to pay attention to details
   d. being good at math

3. Medical records are important for many reasons. Their most important purpose is for legal protection. (T or F)

4. It is acceptable to release medical information to a family member as long as you have written authorization from the patient. (T or F)

5. When charting, you should determine the relevant information and leave out the opinions and incidentals, unless they relate to the patient's medical care. (T or F)

6. Medical filing systems may be based on the alphabet, a numeric system, or by subject. (T or F)

CERTIFICATION CRITERIA CHECKLIST

As you go through your education and training, keep in mind the national certification examination that you will take when you graduate. Each chapter of the textbook and workbook covers a different section of the examination criteria. To keep track of your preparation for the certification examination, turn to the back of this workbook and highlight the following CMA, RMA, or

CMAS certification examination criteria (if you have already highlighted them from a previous chapter, put a check mark by the criteria):

CMA
D.   Professionalism
    4.   Maintaining confidentiality
F.   Medicolegal Guidelines & Requirements
    3.   Documentation/reporting
    4.   Releasing medical information
J.   Records Management

RMA
II.   Administrative Medical Assisting
    C.   Medical Receptionist/Secretarial/Clerical
        5.   Records and chart management

CMAS
4.   Medical Records Management

COMPETENCY ASSESSMENT

Procedure 14-1 Steps for Manual Filing with a Numeric System

Performance Objectives: To demonstrate an understanding of the principles of the numeric filing system. Perform this objective within 15 minutes with a minimum score of 35 points.

Supplies/Equipment: Documents to be filed, dividers with guides, miscellaneous number file section, alphabetic card file and cards, accession journal if needed

Charting/Documentation: Enter appropriate documentation/charting in the box.

_____

_____

_____

_____

Instructor's/Evaluator's Comments and Suggestions:

_____

_____

_____

_____

_____

_____

SKILLS CHECKLIST Procedure 14-1: Steps for Manual Filing with a Numeric System

Name _____

Date _____

No.	Skill	Check #1 20 pts ea	Check #2 10 pts ea	Check #3 5 pts ea	Notes
1	Inspect and index.				
2	Code for filing units.				
3	Write the number in the upper-right corner.				
4	If no number is assigned, check the miscellaneous file. If item is ready to be assigned, make a card and note number, cross out M, and make a chart file.				
5	If there is no card, make up an alphabetic card.				
6	Cross-reference if necessary and file the card properly.				
7	File in ascending order.				
Student's Total Points					
Points Possible		140	70	35	
Final Score (Student's Total Points / Possible Points)					
		Notes			
Start time:					
End time:					
Total time: (15 min goal)					

COMPETENCY ASSESSMENT
Procedure 14-2 Steps for Manual Filing with a Subject Filing System

Performance Objectives: To demonstrate an understanding of the principles of the numeric filing system. Perform this objective within 15 minutes with a minimum score of 35 points.

Supplies/Equipment: Documents to be filed by subject, subject index list or index card filing listing subjects, alphabetic card file and cards

Charting/Documentation: Enter appropriate documentation/charting in the box.

_____

_____

_____

_____

Instructor's/Evaluator's Comments and Suggestions:

_____

_____

_____

_____

_____

_____

SKILLS CHECKLIST Procedure 14-2: Steps for Manual Filing with a Subject Filing System

Name _____

Date _____

No.	Skill	Check #1 20 pts ea	Check #2 10 pts ea	Check #3 5 pts ea	Notes
1	Review the item to find the subject.				
2	Match the subject of the item with an appropriate category.				
3	If neccessary, decide on proper cross-reference.				
4	Underline any subject title on the material.				
5	Write subject title in upper right corner and underline.				
6	Use wavy underline for cross-referencing; use an X as with alphabetic and numeric filing.				
7	Underline the first indexing unit.				
Student's Total Points					
Points Possible		140	70	35	
Final Score (Student's Total Points / Possible Points)					

	Notes
Start time:	
End time:	
Total time: (15 min goal)	

COMPETENCY ASSESSMENT

Procedure 14-3 Correcting a Paper Medical Record

Performance Objectives: To demonstrate the appropriate method to correct an error in a medical chart. Perform this objective within 3 minutes with a minimum score of 25 points.

Supplies/Equipment: Document containing error, document containing correction, red ink pen

Charting/Documentation: Enter appropriate documentation/charting in the box.

_____

_____

_____

_____

Instructor's/Evaluator's Comments and Suggestions:

_____

_____

_____

_____

_____

SKILLS CHECKLIST Procedure 14-3: Correcting a Paper Medical Record

Name _____

Date _____

No.	Skill	Check #1 20 pts ea	Check #2 10 pts ea	Check #3 5 pts ea	Notes
1	Review information on correction of medical records.				
2	Draw single red line through error.				
3	Write in the correct information.				
4	Follow standard clinic protocol (options: make "error" or "correction" notation above error or corrected information).				
5	Initial and date the correction.				
Student's Total Points					
Points Possible		100	50	25	
Final Score (Student's Total Points / Possible Points)					

	Notes
Start time:	
End time:	
Total time: (3 min goal)	

COMPETENCY ASSESSMENT

Procedure 14-4 Correcting an Electronic Medical Record

Performance Objectives: To demonstrate the appropriate method of correction errors in electronic medical records. Perform this objective within 3 minutes with a minimum score of 30 points.

Supplies/Equipment: Computer with screen open to document containing error, document containing correction

Charting/Documentation: Enter appropriate documentation/charting in the box.

_____

_____

_____

_____

Instructor's/Evaluator's Comments and Suggestions:

_____

_____

_____

_____

_____

SKILLS CHECKLIST Procedure 14-4: Correcting an Electronic Medical Record

Name _____

Date _____

No.	Skill	Check #1 20 pts ea	Check #2 10 pts ea	Check #3 5 pts ea	Notes
1	Review information on correcting EMRs.				
2	Set the software to track the area to be corrected.				
3	Line out the error using the dash key.				
4	Key in the correction to be made beside the error.				
5	Follow clinic protocol (option: key in "correction" or "error" near the corrected information/error).				
6	Initial and date the correction.				
Student's Total Points					
Points Possible		120	60	30	
Final Score (Student's Total Points / Possible Points)					

	Notes
Start time:	
End time:	
Total time: (3 min goal)	

COMPETENCY ASSESSMENT

Procedure 14-5 Establishing a Paper Medical Chart for a New Patient

Performance Objectives: To demonstrate an understanding of the principles for establishing a paper medical chart. Perform this objective within 15 minutes with a minimum score of 50 points.

Supplies/Equipment: File folder used in the facility (flip-up or book-style), divider pages used in the facility (SOAP, laboratory reports, HIPAA Information Sheets, etc.), adhesive twin-prong fasteners for divider pages, two-hole punch for twin-prong fasteners, selected tabs to identify folder and divider pages, demographic patient information completed before or at the first appointment

Charting/Documentation: Enter appropriate documentation/charting in the box.

_____

_____

_____

_____

Instructor's/Evaluator's Comments and Suggestions:

_____

_____

_____

_____

_____

SKILLS CHECKLIST Procedure 14-5: Establishing a Paper Medical Chart for a New Patient

Name _____

Date _____

No.	Skill	Check #1 20 pts ea	Check #2 10 pts ea	Check #3 5 pts ea	Notes
1	Assemble all supplies at a desk or table.				
2	Punch holes in the manila file folder and any necessary dividers.				
3	Affix the adhesive twin-prong fasteners.				
4	Assemble the divider pages dictated by the practice and the office policy.				
5	Securely fasten twin-prong fasteners over the divider pages.				
6	Index and code the patient's name according to the filing system to be used.				
7	Affix appropriately labeled tabs to the folder cut.				
8	Transfer demographic data in black ink pen or office demographic divider sheet.				
9	Affix HIPAA required information, read and signed by patient.				
10	Place prepared chart in proper location.				
Student's Total Points					
Points Possible		200	100	50	
Final Score (Student's Total Points / Possible Points)					

	Notes
Start time:	
End time:	
Total time: (15 min goal)	

EVALUATION OF CHAPTER KNOWLEDGE

	Student Self-Evaluation		
Skills	Good	Average	Poor
I can state the reasons for accurately maintaining office files.	_____	_____	_____
I recall common supplies used in medical records management.	_____	_____	_____
I can name and describe basic rules for filing.	_____	_____	_____
I recall steps for filing medical documentation in patient files.	_____	_____	_____
I recall filing procedures for correspondence.	_____	_____	_____
I can state advantages and disadvantages of the alphabetic filing system.	_____	_____	_____
I can distinguish between filing systems, such as alphabetic, numeric, and subject filing.	_____	_____	_____
I understand color-coded filing systems.	_____	_____	_____
I can analyze the purposes of cross-referencing.			
I recall four common documents filed in the patient's medical record.	_____	_____	_____
I can describe computer databases and their usefulness to the ambulatory care setting.	_____	_____	_____
I understand rules of confidentiality when handling patients' medical records.	_____	_____	_____

CHAPTER 15

Written Communications

CHAPTER PRE-TEST

Perform this test without looking at the book. This is just to see how well you have understood and can recall the information in this chapter after you have read it, but before you have completed the workbook exercises. You will not be graded on this portion (other than the grade you give yourself). Justify any "false" answers.

1. The four major letter styles are (circle four):
   a. full block
   b. modified block, standard
   c. facilitated block
   d. simplified block
   e. simplified
   f. modified block, indented

2. The part of a letter that includes a specially designed logo with the address and phone numbers is called the:
   a. salutation
   b. inside address
   c. letterhead
   d. reference heading
   e. enclosure

3. Whenever documents are to be included in a mailed letter, the word *enclosure* should be written out completely and placed one or two lines below the reference initials. (T or F)

4. Envelopes should be addressed using block (uppercase) letters and no punctuation. (T or F)

5. A computerized feature that allows you to send the same letter, although personalized, to many different people using a database is called:

a. word processing letters

b. mail merge

c. database letters

d. merge correspondence

6. E-mail is a casual correspondence method; therefore, spelling and grammar are not important. (T or F)

INTRODUCTION

Written correspondence in the ambulatory care setting has three important functions: it conveys necessary information to patients, other physicians, and health care organizations; it reflects on the professional standards of the office; and it provides permanent legal documentation in the event of any litigation. It is essential that medical assisting students understand the importance of written communication skills. Valuable skills include being able to distinguish between and compose the four major letter styles used in the ambulatory care setting; being able to proofread for spelling, grammar, and content; and being able to describe the significance of accuracy in, and the basic rules of, medical transcription.

PERFORMANCE OBJECTIVES

After successful completion of this chapter you should be able to discuss the purposes and uses of written communication in the ambulatory care setting, identify your responsibilities toward written communication, list major letter styles, compose and create appropriate business letters, use official proofreader's marks when proofing a document/letter, address envelopes according to acceptable postal regulations, use computers for electronic communication and to create mass mailings, and be able to sort and classify incoming mail properly according to your office policies. *The following statements are related to your learning objectives for this chapter. Fill in the blanks in the following paragraph with the appropriate term(s).*

All written communication should be of excellent quality because it (1) _____ on the professionalism of the office. Written documents are (2) _____ legal documents in the event of any litigation. Medical assistants should remember that there is a difference between (3) _____ and business correspondence. It is best to keep business letters to one page, if possible. It is important the business correspondence contain no (4) _____ errors and no words that are used incorrectly. Keep a dictionary handy for reference as needed. Computerized (5) _____ tools are not infallible and should be relied on with caution. Components of a business letter include the (6) _____ line, (7) _____ address, (8) _____, (9) _____ line, (10) _____ of the letter, (11) _____ closing, keyed (12) _____, and (13) _____ initials. Business letters may also include a (14) _____ notation, (15) _____ notation, (16) _____, and continuation (17) _____ heading. (18) _____ marks are a universally accepted method of marking documents to highlight suggested changes, errors, and inaccuracies. There are many different styles of letters. The most widely accepted styles in a business setting are the (19) _____, (20) _____, and (21) _____. Postal preferences for envelopes have been established to create a quicker, more efficient, and more reliable mail delivery system, especially with the use of (22) _____ character readers. Among the suggestions are the elimination of all (23) _____, use of a uniform (24) _____ margin, preference toward all (25) _____ letters, and the absence of all marks in the (26) _____ of the envelope. The zip code should contain all (27) _____ numbers. Mail (28) _____ is an excellent use of computers in the medical office that eliminates the need to rekey the same letter many times when sent to a variety of people, and yet allows the letter to be personalized for each recipient. When handling incoming mail, the first step is to (29) _____ it into different categories. Then the mail should be (30) _____ with the date received and checked for a return (31) _____. Then attach the letter/document to the (32) _____ and either route it appropriately, attach supporting documentation, or reply as promptly as possible.

VOCABULARY BUILDER

Fill in the blanks in the passage below with the correct vocabulary terms.

bond paper	optical character reader (OCR)
full block letter	simplified letter
keyed	voice recognition technology (VRT)
mail merge	watermark
medical transcription	Zip+4
modified block letter	

There are four major types of letters that medical assistants commonly write. Of these, the (1) _____ is the most time-efficient, because it does not use excessive tab indentations for the address, complimentary close, or keyed signature. In the (2) _____, all lines begin at the left margin with the exception of the date line, complimentary closure, and keyed signature. Medical assistants may choose to use the (3) _____, the style of letter recommended by the Administrative Management Society. In this style, all lines are (4) _____, or input by keystroke, flush with the left margin. When selecting paper supplies, the medical assistant should choose (5) _____ with a (6) _____, or image imprinted during the papermaking process that is visible when a sheet is held up to the light. When preparing letters for outgoing shipments, it is important for the medical assistant to pay attention to several factors, including addresses. Medical assistants should machine print addresses (including the (7) _____ code) with a uniform left-hand margin so that the addresses can be read by the U.S. Postal Service's (8) _____.

One of the most utilized aspects of written communication in the clinic is the management of the patient records, which are processed in the arena of (9) _____. One of the latest technical advances in this area is (10) _____, by which physicians speak into a microphone that translates spoken words into a typed report via the computer. This new method can cut down on errors and aid medical assistants in maintaining confidentiality and protecting the privacy of patients in the process of medical documentation.

LEARNING REVIEW

1. Identify the letter style in Figure 15-1. _____

2. Proofread the letter in Figure 15-1, correcting all errors by inserting the proper proofreader's marks. Make your marks directly onto the text. Consult your textbook for a list of common proofreader's marks. Refer to a medical dictionary, if necessary.

3. To practice your skills of medical transcription, record the content of the letter in Figure 15-1 by speaking into a tape recorder. Play back the tape and transcribe the letter accurately on a sheet of stationery using the standard modified block style.

JAMES CARTER, MD, NEUROLOGY

Metropolitan University Medical Center, 8280 Wright Avenue, Northborough, OH 12382

February 2, 20XX

Elizabeth Kind, M.D
Inner City Health Care
The Offices of Lewis & King, MD
2501 Center Street
Nrothborough, OH 12345

RE: MARGARET THOMAS

Dear Dr. King:

Thank you for refering Margaret Thomas to my neurological practice. Margaret come to you recently as a new patient for a comprehensive physical examination to evaluate troubling symptoms she had been experiencing for several months. Margaret notices symtoms of tremor, difficulty walking, defective judgement, and hot flushes; she is not able to poinpoint the exac ttime symptoms began. Your physical examination suggested the possible diagnoisis of parkingson's Disease. Margaret presented today for a complete nuerological evaluation.

Figure 15-1

c. return address

d. closing remark (such as: "Sincerely")

e. the recipient's name, title, and address

3. When addressing an envelope, the proper way to list the state is:

a. to write it out completely

b. to abbreviate it using at least the first four letters

c. to capitalize it using the official two-letter abbreviation

d. any of the above as long as it is in uppercase letters and is written clearly

4. URL means:

a. Universal Return (address) Locator

b. Uniform Resource Locator

c. Universal Readers Limitation

d. Uniform Registered Locator

CASE STUDY

Ellen Armstrong, CMA, enjoys working on correspondence for Drs. Lewis and King and takes pride in her written communication skills. As an ongoing project, office manager Marilyn Johnson, CMA, asks Ellen to make suggestions for updating and revising the style manual used in the medical office for written communication guidelines. Ellen suggests the addition of a section in the style manual to discuss bias in language. Bias-free language is sensitive in applying labels to individuals or groups and uses sex-specific words and pronouns appropriately. For example, dementia is used instead of crazy or senile. Instead of using layman, consider using layperson. Apply he or she only in sex-specific usage. Marilyn and the physician–employers ask Ellen to implement the addition to the style manual.

Discuss the following:
1. Why is bias-free language an important consideration in written communications for the ambulatory care setting?
2. List other examples of biased language and give suggestions for bias-free alternatives.

SELF-ASSESSMENT

In your written communications, are you able to express yourself accurately and concisely? Able to communicate ideas effectively? Capable of proofreading and editing for content? Use this simple self-assessment to gauge your comfort and proficiency in written communications by identifying strengths and pinpointing any weak areas that could use improvement.

For each statement below, circle the corresponding letter to the response that best describes you.

1. When writing a letter, I generally feel:

a. confident. I communicate effectively on the page and enjoy writing letters.

b. at ease. My written communication skills are acceptable.

c. uncomfortable. I would rather communicate verbally than through writing.

2. As far as content goes, when I am given the required information and asked to compose a letter, I:

   a. almost always understand exactly what I am being asked to communicate and am able to convey it precisely in letter form

   b. generally understand what I am being asked to communicate, but sometimes have to fine-tune my letters

   c. often have trouble understanding what I am being asked to communicate and usually have to go back and ask questions about the letter's content

3. In general, when choosing words for written correspondence, I feel:

   a. secure about my ability to select appropriate language and use medical terminology accurately

   b. pretty confident, although my general vocabulary and knowledge of medical terminology could use some improvement

   c. frustrated; I always seem to confuse words and medical terms no matter how hard I try not to

4. As far as spelling goes, I am:

   a. a top-notch speller; I always keep both a standard and medical dictionary on hand for the words I am not sure of.

   b. an adequate speller; sometimes I confuse a word here or there; I always have to proofread carefully for spelling errors

   c. a below-par speller; my letters are always littered with misspellings and someone else has to proofread my work

5. Grammatically speaking, I am:

   a. above average; I routinely find mistakes in my colleagues' work

   b. passable; I make minor mistakes but usually catch them while proofreading

   c. hopeless; people find mistakes in my work even after I have checked it twice

6. Regarding proofreader's marks, I am:

   a. highly capable of proofreading my work; if colleagues need someone to proof their work, I am first on their list

   b. an okay proofreader; I occasionally overlook a mistake, but nobody's perfect

   c. frightened; proofreading marks are just a bunch of meaningless squiggles to me

7. How would you describe your formatting skills?

   a. Exemplary. I understand all basic letter forms, and all of my letters are rigorously formatted according to correct specifications.

   b. Satisfactory. Every so often, I confuse styles or forget an annotation; but in general, all my letters are formatted correctly.

   c. Fair to nonexistent. I have trouble understanding why every letter has to be so formally constructed.

8. When adhering to office style guidelines, I:

   a. always follow the guidelines

   b. usually have no problem sticking to style guidelines; when I make a mistake, it is a rare event

   c. need improvement; my letters are frequently littered with style inconsistencies, and I do not understand the need for an office style as long as each letter is written with accurate information

9. If you had to rate your transcription skills, you would describe them as:

   a. impeccable. I make few errors and use critical thinking skills to problem-solve trouble spots before giving up and asking for help.

   b. sufficient. What I do not understand I automatically flag and ask for clarification.

   c. not as good as they should be. I hate trying to enter data from a taped voice; it is a frustrating experience.

10. Overall, I think of writing letters in the health care environment as:

    a. one of my strong suits

    b. a task that I am able to accomplish, just not one I particularly enjoy

    c. a necessary evil

Scoring: If your answers were mostly A responses, you have strong written communications skills and enjoy writing letters. If your responses were mostly Bs, your written communications skills are good but could stand some improvement. Try reviewing pertinent information in this chapter to strengthen areas that need it. If your answers were mostly Cs, you need to work on your written communication skills. Volunteer to take on as many written correspondence assignments as you can—practice may help you overcome your apprehension about writing letters and will almost certainly raise the quality of your work.

CHAPTER POST-TEST

This is similar to the Pre-Test. Perform this test without looking at the book. This is just to see how well you have understood and can recall the information presented in this chapter after you have studied it and completed the workbook exercises. You will not be graded on this portion (other than the grade you give yourself), but this is an excellent preparation for your instructor's test. You may use this Post-Test to determine what areas you need to study more. Justify any "false" answers.

1. The most commonly used of the four major letter styles in the ambulatory care setting is:

   a. full block

   b. modified block, standard

   c. facilitated block, indented

   d. simplified

2. The part of a letter that includes the return address and perhaps a logo is the:

   a. salutation

   b. inside address

   c. letterhead

   d. reference heading

   e. enclosure

3. Whenever documents are to be included in a mailed letter, the word *enclosure* should be indicated by:

   a. Enclosures

   b. Enc.

   c. 1 Enc.

   d. 2 enclosures

   e. Enclosure (2)

   f. any of the above

4. Envelopes should be addressed using a combination of uppercase and lowercase letters and with the proper punctuation. (T or F)

5. When it is desirable to send the same letter, although personalized, to many different people, a computerized feature that can be used is called:

   a. word processing letters

   b. mail merge

   c. database letters

   d. merge correspondence

6. E-mail may be used as a type of business correspondence method and is subject to the same proper use of written language as traditional mail. (T or F)

CERTIFICATION CRITERIA CHECKLIST

As you go through your education and training, keep in mind the national certification examination that you will take when you graduate. Each chapter of the textbook and workbook covers a different section of the examination criteria. To keep track of your preparation for the certification examination turn to the back of this workbook and highlight the following CMA, RMA, or CMAS certification examination criteria (if you have already highlighted them from a previous chapter, put a check mark by the criteria):

CMA
A. Medical Terminology
    2.   Uses of terminology
E. Communication
    7.   Receiving, organizing, prioritizing and transmitting information
    9.   Fundamental writing skills

G. Data Entry
    2. Formats
    3. Proofreading
H. Equipment
    1. Equipment operation
I. Computer Concepts
    3. Computer applications
K. Screening and Processing Mail

RMA
I. General Medical Assisting Knowledge
    B. Medical Terminology
        4. Spelling
II. Administrative Medical Assisting
    C. Medical Receptionist/Secretary/Clerical
        4. (Oral and) Written communication

CMAS
8. Medical Office Management
    • Office communications

COMPETENCY ASSESSMENT
Procedure 15-1 Preparing and Composing Business Correspondence Using All Components (Computerized Approach)

Performance Objectives: To prepare and compose a final copy letter using appropriate language and letter style to convey a clear and accurate message to the recipient. Perform this objective within 20 minutes with a minimum score of 100 points.

Supplies/Equipment: Computer and printer, printed letterhead and plain second sheet, dictionary (medical and standard), thesaurus, style resource

Charting/Documentation: Enter appropriate documentation/charting in the box.

_____

_____

_____

_____

Instructor's/Evaluator's Comments and Suggestions:

_____

_____

_____

_____

_____

SKILLS CHECKLIST Procedure 15-1: Preparing and Composing Business Correspondence Using All Components (Computerized Approach)

Name _____

Date _____

No.	Skill	Check #1 20 pts ea	Check #2 10 pts ea	Check #3 5 pts ea	Notes
1	Organize the key points in a logical sequence.				
2	Set margins and other layout parameters, choose and set fonts. Save the document.				
3	Compose a rough outline of the letter.				
4	Use easily understood language. State the reason for the letter in the first paragraph and encourage action in the last paragraph.				
5	Read the draft for errors. Use appropriate reference materials. Read again for content. Save it. Print it out or access it later for a third check.				
6	Choose the format that is customary for your situation.				
7	Key in the date on line 15 or two to three lines below the letterhead.				
8	Key in the recipient's name and address flush with the left margin beginning on line 20.				
9	On the second line below the recipient's address, key the salutation flush with the left margin. Place a colon after the salutation unless using open punctuation.				
10	Key the subject of the letter on the second line below the salutation flush with the left margin.				
11	Begin the body of the letter on the second line below the salutation or subject line. Single space within paragraphs, and double space between paragraphs.				
12	Key the complimentary closure on the second line below the body of the letter. Capitalize only the first letter of the first word of the complimentary closure.				
13	Key in the signature four to six lines below the closure.				

No.	Skill	Check #1 20 pts ea	Check #2 10 pts ea	Check #3 5 pts ea	Notes
14	If reference initials are used, key the initials two lines below the keyed signature.				
15	Key the enclosure or copy notation one or two lines below the reference initials.				
16	Proofread the document and make corrections as necessary.				
17	Save the document again and print two copies.				
18	Prepare the envelope. Place the envelope flap over the letter and attach it with a clip. Attach it to the patient chart if appropriate.				
19	Place the letter on the physician's desk for review and signature.				
20	File a copy of the letter in an appropriate filing system.				
Student's Total Points					
Points Possible		400	200	100	
Final Score (Student's Total Points / Possible Points)					
		Notes			
Start time:					
End time:					
Total time: (20 min goal)					

COMPETENCY ASSESSMENT

Procedure 15-2 Addressing Envelopes According to United States Postal Regulations

Performance Objectives: To address envelopes according to U.S. Postal Service regulations to ensure timely delivery. Perform this objective within 5 minutes with a minimum score of 25 points.

Supplies/Equipment: Computer and printer with envelope tray, envelopes, address labels, U.S. Postal Service Publication 221, Addressing for Success

Charting/Documentation: Enter appropriate documentation/charting in the box.

_____

_____

_____

_____

Instructor's/Evaluator's Comments and Suggestions:

_____

_____

_____

_____

_____

SKILLS CHECKLIST Procedure 15-2: Addressing Envelopes According to United States Postal Regulations

Name _____

Date _____

No.	Skill	Check #1 20 pts ea	Check #2 10 pts ea	Check #3 5 pts ea	Notes
1	Select the envelope format from the software program, or use labels.				
2	Place the address within the proper area as directed by the U.S. postal regulations.				
3	Key the address in uppercase letters. Maintain a uniform left margin. Eliminate all punctuation except the hyphen in the zip code. Leave one space between the city and the two-character state abbreviation and the zip code.				
4	If not using preprinted envelopes, key the return address in upper-case letters in the upper left corner: name on the first line; address on the second; and city, state, and zip code on the third line.				
5	Proofread the envelope, make corrections as necessary.				
Student's Total Points					
Points Possible		100	50	25	
Final Score (Student's Total Points / Possible Points)					

	Notes
Start time:	
End time:	
Total time: (5 min goal)	

COMPETENCY ASSESSMENT

Procedure 15-3 Folding Letters for Standard Envelopes

Performance Objectives: To fold and insert letters into envelopes so that the letters fit properly in the envelopes. Perform this objective within 2 minutes with a minimum score of 15 points.

Supplies/Equipment: Letters to be mailed, number 6¾ envelope, number 10 envelope, window envelope

Charting/Documentation: Enter appropriate documentation/charting in the box.

_____

_____

_____

_____

Instructor's/Evaluator's Comments and Suggestions:

_____

_____

_____

_____

_____

SKILLS CHECKLIST Procedure 15-3: Folding Letters for Standard Envelopes

Name _____

Date _____

No.	Skill	Check #1 20 pts ea	Check #2 10 pts ea	Check #3 5 pts ea	Notes
1	Fold letter to fit into a number 6¾ envelope.				
2	Fold letter to fit into a number 10 envelope.				
3	Fold letter to fit into a window envelope.				
Student's Total Points					
Points Possible		60	30	15	
Final Score (Student's Total Points / Possible Points)					

	Notes
Start time:	
End time:	
Total time: (2 min goal)	

COMPETENCY ASSESSMENT
Procedure 15-4 Creating a Mass Mailing Using Mail Merge

Performance Objectives: To create a mass mailing using the computer's Mail Merge Helper feature contained within Microsoft® Word. Perform this objective within 15 minutes with a minimum score of 20 points.

Supplies/Equipment: Computer and printer, composed correspondence keyed and saved as a Word document, a developed data source

Charting/Documentation: Enter appropriate documentation/charting in the box.

_____

_____

_____

_____

Instructor's/Evaluator's Comments and Suggestions:

_____

_____

_____

_____

_____

_____

SKILLS CHECKLIST Procedure 15-4: Creating a Mass Mailing Using Mail Merge

Name _____

Date _____

No.	Skill	Check #1 20 pts ea	Check #2 10 pts ea	Check #3 5 pts ea	Notes
1	Compose and type the document.				
2	Develop a data source.				
3	Insert merge fields into the main document.				
4	Send the merged document to the output device (printer).				
Student's Total Points					
Points Possible		80	40	20	
Final Score (Student's Total Points / Possible Points)					

	Notes
Start time:	
End time:	
Total time: (15 min goal)	

COMPETENCY ASSESSMENT

Procedure 15-5 Preparing Outgoing Mail According to United States Postal Regulations

Performance Objectives: To prepare outgoing mail for expeditious delivery. Perform this objective within 15 minutes with a minimum score of 20 points.

Supplies/Equipment: Manual or electronic scale, postage meter or stamps, envelope or package to be mailed

Charting/Documentation: Enter appropriate documentation/charting in the box.

_____

_____

_____

_____

Instructor's/Evaluator's Comments and Suggestions:

_____

_____

_____

_____

_____

_____

SKILLS CHECKLIST Procedure 15-5: Preparing Outgoing Mail According to United States Postal Regulations

Name _____

Date _____

No.	Skill	Check #1 20 pts ea	Check #2 10 pts ea	Check #3 5 pts ea	Notes
1	Sort the mail according to postal class.				
2	Weigh the item to be mailed.				
3	Affix the appropriate postage.				
4	Place item(s) in outgoing mail, or deliver to post office.				
Student's Total Points					
Points Possible		80	40	20	
Final Score (Student's Total Points / Possible Points)					

	Notes
Start time:	
End time:	
Total time: (15 min goal)	

COMPETENCY ASSESSMENT
Procedure 15-6 Preparing, Sending, and Receiving a Fax

Performance Objectives: To send and receive information quickly and accurately by fax (facsimile). Perform this objective within 15 minutes with a minimum score of 35 points.

Supplies/Equipment: Fax machine, telephone

Charting/Documentation: Enter appropriate documentation/charting in the box.

_____

_____

_____

_____

Instructor's/Evaluator's Comments and Suggestions:

_____

_____

_____

_____

_____

_____

SKILLS CHECKLIST Procedure 15-6: Preparing, Sending, and Receiving a Fax

Name _____

Date _____

No.	Skill	Check #1 20 pts ea	Check #2 10 pts ea	Check #3 5 pts ea	Notes
1	Prepare a cover sheet.				
2	Place the document according to machine instructions.				
3	Dial the telephone number of the receiver.				
4	After document passes through, press button requesting a receipt.				
5	Remove the document and call recipient to verify delivery.				
6	To receive: Turn on fax machine, and check to see that phone line is available.				
7	Remove document from machine after it is received and deliver to addressee.				
Student's Total Points					
Points Possible		140	70	35	
Final Score (Student's Total Points / Possible Points)					

	Notes
Start time:	
End time:	
Total time: (15 min goal)	

EVALUATION OF CHAPTER KNOWLEDGE

Skills	Student Self-Evaluation		
	Good	Average	Poor
I understand the importance of written correspondence in the professional health care setting.	____	____	____
I understand the four basic types of letters medical assistants usually write and how to compose them.	____	____	____
I can correctly spell difficult and commonly misspelled and misused words.	____	____	____
I can use medical terminology appropriately.	____	____	____
I frequently consult standard and medical dictionaries and references when writing.	____	____	____
I understand and can apply proofreader's marks.	____	____	____
I understand the components of business letters, (e.g., date line, salutation, body of letter, reference initials, postscripts, etc.).	____	____	____
I can identify and use supplies for written communications.	____	____	____
I can accurately process incoming and outgoing mail and packages according to U.S. postal regulations.	____	____	____
I understand how to use new technologies designed for written communications (e.g., facsimile machines, modems).	____	____	____
I comprehend the importance of medical transcription.	____	____	____
I am able to recall the basic tools of medical transcription.	____	____	____
I am sensitive to bias in language and can develop strategies for bias-free writing.	____	____	____
I can apply computer concepts to office procedures.	____	____	____
I can adapt communication to individuals' abilities to understand.	____	____	____

CHAPTER 16

Transcription

CHAPTER PRE-TEST

Perform this test without looking at the book. This is just to see how well you have understood and can recall the information in this chapter after you have read it, but before you have completed the workbook exercises. You will not be graded on this portion (other than the grade you give yourself). Justify any "false" answers.

1. Medical transcriptionists must have years of experience before they can do well in the field. (T or F)

2. Anyone who has computer abilities and can spell well can perform medical transcription well. (T or F)

3. Medical documents are only for the clinic and physician who generated them, so they are called "internal documents." (T or F)

4. Medical transcription is a profession that has not really undergone many changes in the last decade or so. (T or F)

5. If a medical transcriptionist cannot hear the word the dictator is saying, it is best to leave the space blank. (T or F)

6. Even though medical transcriptionists work within the medical field, because they often work alone, they do not need to be concerned with Health Insurance Portability and Accountability Act (HIPAA) regulations. (T or F)

INTRODUCTION

Many medical offices have transcription services available in the office for the physician to dictate the medical record. Those able to provide transcription services are highly skilled professionals who are in demand for their skills. The medical assistant who is able to provide these skills is in high demand. Medical transcription involves a knowledge of the equipment, including transcription machines and computers for word processing, the use of correct medical terminology for the many types of records used in the office, the ability to format documents, and good proofreading skills. The correct usage of grammar, spelling, and punctuation aids the medical assistant in demonstrating good transcription skills.

PERFORMANCE OBJECTIVES

Your career as a medical assistant may or may not include transcription, but it will certainly include medical documents. Transcription is all about medical documents such as chart notes, operative reports, history and physical examination reports, discharge summaries, emergency room summaries, radiology and pathology reports, and consultation reports, as well letters to patients and other physicians. Taking a course in transcription incorporates lessons learned in medical terminology, anatomy and physiology, pathology, word processing, English, spelling, sentence structure, grammar, proofreading, and punctuation. There is perhaps no other course that encompasses so many other course lessons. Other lessons well learned in medical transcription are less objective; for example, the lessons of striving for quality, neatness, completeness, and accuracy. Medical records are legal documents, thus perfection is the goal. Many physicians rely on the medical transcriptionist to produce perfect documents, and with this responsibility comes trust. When physicians trust that the documents are correct and accurate, they will often sign them without thoroughly proofreading them. A transcriptionist who betrays that trust puts the physician at risk legally.

Many medical clinics employ transcriptionists in the office, whereas others contract their transcription services. As a transcriptionist, you may choose to be self-employed, a contracted employee, or an employee of the clinic. Within those parameters, the actual transcription work may be performed in-house or at a remote site. The documents may be printed and brought into the office, sent in electronically for printing within the office, or, in the case of EMRs (electronic medical records), the data may be entered directly into the computer and saved in the patient's electronic chart. *The following statements are related to your learning objectives for this chapter. Fill in the blanks in the following paragraph with the appropriate term(s).*

Medical transcription is all about medical (1) _____. Medical transcriptionists must have a good working knowledge about medical (2) _____,

anatomy and (3) _____, disease processes (4)_____

and word processing. They must know English, (5) _____,

(6) _____, (7) _____, and

(8) _____. Medical documents are (9)_____

documents; therefore, the transcriptionist must strive for (10) _____,

(11) _____, (12) _____, and

(13) _____.

VOCABULARY BUILDER

Find the words below that are misspelled; circle them, and then correctly spell them in the spaces provided. Then insert the correct vocabulary terms from the list that best fit the descriptions below.

athentication	discharge summary	priveliged
autapsy report	electronic	progress notes
chart notes	gross examination	proofreading
chief complaint	HIPAA	quality assurance
confidentility	history and physical	review of symptoms
consultation reports	JCAHO	risk management
continuing education	magnetic tape	transcriber
correspondence	medical transcriptionist	

current   microscopic examination   turnaround time

digital speech standard   old   voice recognition system

digitaly processed dictation   patholigy   waveform audio

_____   _____   _____

_____   _____   _____

_____   _____

1. A professional who uses word processing formats to transcribe medical records, notes, letters, and documents is called a _____.

2. The part of the pathology report that describes the size and shape of a biopsy is called a _____.

3. The part of patients' hospital records that describe their entire hospital stay, progress, and condition on release is called a _____.

4. The part of the patient's medical record that contains information related to the main reason for the encounter, as well as a synopsis of the patient's previous medical information, is called the _____.

5. Reports such as History and Physicals that should be completed within 24 hours are called _____ reports.

6. A type of signature that may use various computer key entries as identification is referred to as _____.

7. The process of converting audio sound into a string of computer language is called _____ _____.

8. A medical report generated to describe the examinations of tissues or cells obtained through a surgery or medical procedure is the _____ report.

9. Reports that may be completed up to 71 hours after the event are referred to as _____ _____ reports.

Define the following terms:

1. American Association for Medical Transcription

_____

_____

2. Consultation report

_____

_____

3. Digital speech standard

_____

_____

4. Editing

_____

_____

5. Flag

_____

_____

6. Home-based medical transcriptionists

_____

_____

7. Turnaround time

_____

_____

8. Digital dictation

_____

_____

LEARNING REVIEW

1. A. List five attributes of the medical transcriptionist under each of the two major categories.

  (1) Personal attributes

    a. _____

    b. _____

    c. _____

    d. _____

    e. _____

  (2) Acquired skills developed

    a. _____

    b. _____

    c. _____

    d. _____

    e. _____

  B. Describe how the transcription machine (transcriber) differs from a simple audio recorder.

_____

_____

_____

C. Correct the following paragraph:

her past medical history is postivie for the usual childhood diseases and the births of to children following normal pregnancies she has a negative pasts urgical history. she has no allergies To medications and takes tylenol for occasional headashes. She is married and has to children ages 3 and 12 months. She does not smoke or drink

D. Give two examples of each type of turnaround time report and the time of the turnaround.

STAT: (1) _____

           (2) _____

Current: (1) _____

           (2) _____

Old: (1) _____

           (2) _____

2. The American Association for Medical Transcription (AAMT) began in _____.
   a. 1850
   b. 1902
   c. 1978
   d. 2000

3. Which of the following is *not* a requirement for success in the field of medical transcription?
   a. experience in the medical field
   b. keyboarding skills of 60 to 80 words per minute
   c. understanding of human anatomy
   d. knowledge of drug names and their uses

4. To take the CMT examination, the transcriptionist must have a minimum of _____ years performing medical transcription.
   a. 1
   b. 2
   c. 5
   d. 10

5. CMT recertification is accomplished through continuing education with the purpose of maintaining competency and must be completed every _____ years.
   a. 2
   b. 3
   c. 5
   d. 10

6. Radiology, pathology, and laboratory reports are usually termed as _____ to indicate the need for immediate turnaround.

   a. ASAP

   b. current

   c. old

   d. STAT

CERTIFICATION REVIEW

These questions are designed to mimic the certification examinations. You can use these questions like a small "Certification Examination Study Guide," but this is not meant to take the place of the more extensive study guides. Use this portion to determine in what areas to concentrate your efforts when studying for the certification examination. Justify any "false" answers.

1. Medical records are documents governed by laws and may be subpoenaed for review by various courts. (T or F)

2. The medical report may play a major role in substantiating injury or a malpractice claim. (T or F)

3. Joint Commission on Accreditation of Healthcare Organizations (JCAHO) allows 36 hours from admission for a history and physical report to be dictated, transcribed, and filed into the patient's medical record. (T or F)

4. When transcribing radiology or imaging reports, the date of service should be used rather than the date of dictation. (T or F)

5. Electronic signatures on medical documents are allowed by both Medicare and JCAHO. (T or F)

CASE STUDY

You are transcribing a report when you notice it is a report about your neighbor. The report states that the tests run for multiple sclerosis are positive. You had just spoken to your neighbor yesterday and she was concerned that she hadn't heard from her physician and was wondering about the results of her tests. What should you do?

SELF-ASSESSMENT

1. Access the AAMT Web site at http://www.aamt.org and click on "Certification," then "Candidate's Guide," then the "Sample Medical Transcription Related Knowledge Questions."

   A. Answer the questions to the best of your ability.

   B. Check your answers to see how well you were able to answer the questions correctly.

   C. Which transcription skills listed in the textbook were tested within these questions?

2. Do you think you would enjoy working as a transcriptionist? What about the profession appeals to you? What about the profession does not appeal to you?

CHAPTER POST-TEST

This is similar to the Pre-Test. Perform this test without looking at the book. This is just to see how well you have understood and can recall the information in this chapter after you studied it and completed the workbook exercises. You will not be graded on this portion (other than the grade you give yourself), but this is an excellent preparation for your instructor's test. You may use this Post-Test to determine what areas you need to study more. Justify any "false" answers.

1. Medical transcriptionists can do well even without a lot of experience if they are committed to exactness and quality work. (T or F)

2. Medical transcription is a job for people with good computer abilities, word processing speed; who have excellent spelling, grammar, and punctuation skills; and who care enough to do the best job possible. (T or F)

3. Medical documents are not only for the clinic and physician who generated them, they are also legal documents used by many professionals. (T or F)

4. Medical transcription is a profession that has undergone numerous changes in the last decade or so. (T or F)

5. If a medical transcriptionist cannot hear the word the dictator is saying, it is best to leave the space blank. (T or F)

6. Because medical transcriptionists work within the medical field with medical information, they need to be concerned with HIPAA regulations. (T or F)

CERTIFICATION CRITERIA CHECKLIST

As you go through your education and training, keep in mind the national certification examination that you will take when you graduate. Each chapter of the textbook and workbook covers a different section of the examination criteria. To keep track of your preparation for the certification examination, turn to the back of this workbook and highlight the following CMA, RMA, or CMAS certification examination criteria (if you have already highlighted them from a previous chapter, put a check mark by the criteria):

CMA
A. Medical Terminology
    2. Uses of terminology
F. Medicolegal Guidelines & Requirements
    2. Legislation
G. Data Entry
I. Computer Concepts
    3. Computer applications

RMA
I. General Medical Assisting Knowledge
    B. Medical Terminology
        4. Spelling
II. Administrative Medical Assisting
    C. Medical Receptionist/Secretary/Clerical
        1. Terminology
        4. (Oral and) Written communication
        6. Transcription and dictation
        8. Computer applications

CMAS
1. Medical Assisting Foundation
   - Medical terminology
3. Medical Office Clerical Assisting
   - Communication

EVALUATION OF CHAPTER KNOWLEDGE

Skills	Student Self-Evaluation		
	Good	Average	Poor
I recognize emergency situations.	_____	_____	_____
I can explain the work of the medical transcriptionists, including attributes needed and career opportunities.	_____	_____	_____
I can describe the CMT certification process and membership in AAMT.	_____	_____	_____
I can discuss the proper ways to make corrections.	_____	_____	_____
I can describe the process of flagging.	_____	_____	_____
I can differentiate between the many types of records found in the medical office.	_____	_____	_____
I can describe turnaround time and its importance.	_____	_____	_____
I can discuss ethical and legal issues surrounding medical transcription.	_____	_____	_____

CHAPTER 17

Daily Financial Practices

CHAPTER PRE-TEST

Perform this test without looking at the book. This is just to see how well you have understood and can recall the information in this chapter after you have read it, but before you have completed the workbook exercises. You will not be graded on this portion (other than the grade you give yourself). Justify any "false" answers.

1. The management of the business details of the practice usually falls to the medical assisting staff. (T or F)

2. Every patient, regardless of insurance coverage, should be charged the same fee for the same service. (T or F)

3. You should discourage the use of credit/debit cards for medical bills. (T or F)

4. Purchase orders are to be written up when the purchase arrives. (T or F)

5. Petty cash is available for authorized use when the purchase is minor or unexpected and when a check is not necessary. (T or F)

INTRODUCTION

Ambulatory care settings depend on sound financial practices to thrive, grow, and continue to provide good patient care. To that end, medical assistants should strive to understand basic accounting and bookkeeping terms, forms, principles, and both computerized and manual systems related to these financial activities. Medical assistants should be prepared to handle a variety of financial tasks, including procedures related to accounts receivable, accounts payable, patient billing, banking, checking accounts, purchasing, and petty cash systems.

PERFORMANCE OBJECTIVES

After successful completion of this chapter you will be able to explain the importance of good communication when explaining patient fees. You will have some ideas of available options for credit arrangements for your patients and will be able to recognize when adjustments are warranted. You will be able to differentiate between manual and computerized bookkeeping systems, describe the pegboard system, and state the advantages and disadvantages of computerized book-keeping systems. Another performance objective of this chapter is to help you be aware of and establish good working habits when working with financial records. You will be able to describe information found on and uses for the encounter form. You will be able to demonstrate a knowledge of banking procedures, including types of accounts and services, and show proficiency in preparing deposits, checks, and patient receipts and reconciling accounts. You also will be able to describe month-end activities. *The following statements are related to your learning objectives for this chapter. Fill in the blanks in the following paragraph with the appropriate term(s).*

Accounts (1) _____ are all the fees that patients owe to the practice for services rendered, and accounts (2) _____ are the accounts the practice owes to suppliers for supplies, services, and so forth. When explaining fees to a patient, it is best if the patient knows what to expect before the treatment. Ideally, this should be in (3) _____. The documentation of this discussion with Medicare and Medicaid patients is on a form called the (4) _____, or (5) _____ for short. An (6) _____ to a fee may be warranted for hardship cases, but remember, the same offer must be available to all patients. Patients should be encouraged to use (7) _____ or (8) _____ payments, if those payment methods are handy for them. A(n) (9) _____ form is a document that goes with the patient throughout their visit and includes all the billing information on it. The traditional (10) _____ system of tracking the day's financial activities is quickly being replaced by (11) _____ methods. There are distinct advantages and disadvantages of either method. Occasionally, there is a need for small amounts of cash for minor and unexpected expenses such as a postage due package, coffee or tea for the office, and miscellaneous other needs. This name for this reserve of cash for those purposes is called (12) _____.

VOCABULARY BUILDER

Find the words below that are misspelled; circle them, and then correctly spell them in the spaces provided.

accounts payible	day sheet	notary
accounts recievable	debit	payee
adjustments	dispursements	pegboard system
balance	encounter form	petty cash
cashier's check	guaranter	posting
certified check	leadger	traveler's check
credit	money market account	voucher check

_____   _____   _____

_____   _____

A. *Identify the following financial forms used in the ambulatory care setting.*

_____ 1. Used to records individual cash transactions for minor or unexpected expenses

_____ 2. Record of charges, payments, and adjustments for individual patients and/or family members

_____ 3. A record of daily patient transactions used in conjunction with pegboard systems

_____ 4. Record of services supplied and the charges and payments for those services; functions as a billing form for insurance reimbursement

B. *Identify the correct financial term or function for each definition.*

_____ 1. Agencies that manage many private insurance plans and government-sponsored programs

_____ 2. Small cash sum kept on hand in the office for minor or unexpected expenses

_____ 3. Abbreviation for *received on account*

_____ 4. Decreases the balance due

_____ 5. The amount insurance requires patients to pay at the time of services

_____ 6. A term for paper money

_____ 7. A synonym for *charge slip*

_____ 8. The acceptable abbreviation for *usual, customary, and reasonable* when referring to physician charges

_____ 9. As a noun, this term denotes "the amount owed"; as a verb, the term means "to verify posting accuracy"

_____ 10. Accounting function that describes the act of recording financial transactions into bookkeeping or accounting systems

_____ 11. An increase or decrease to a patient account not due to charges incurred or payments received

_____ 12. Accounting system that consists of day sheets, ledger cards, charge slips, and receipt forms; all forms have matching columns that align and are held in place when the system is in use

_____ 13. Sum owed by a business for services or goods received

_____ 14. Sum owed to a business for services or goods supplied

LEARNING REVIEW

1. Identify two work guidelines and six habits essential to creating and maintaining accurate financial records.

   A. Guidelines:

       (1) _____

       (2) _____

   B. Good work habits:

       (1) _____

       (2) _____

       (3) _____

       (4) _____

       (5) _____

       (6) _____

2. A. The checking account is the account most often used by medical assistants in the ambulatory care setting. Checking accounts are accounts that allow depositors to write checks against money placed in the account. Identify seven of the nine features that may be a part of the checking account.

       (1) _____   (5) _____

       (2) _____   (6) _____

       (3) _____   (7) _____

       (4) _____

   B. Administrative medical assistant Karen Ritter is responsible for assisting the office manager and accountant in performing accounts payable activities for Inner City Health Care. On September 4, she receives a $323.45 bill from RJ Medical Supply Company for blood pressure equipment the office received on August 30. Noting that the company demands payment within 30 days of billing, Karen writes a check disbursing funds to the company on September 15. The balance in the office's checking account before this check is written equals $2,610.00. Using this information, write out the check and stub below (Figure 17-1). Karen will submit the check to Susan Rice, M.D., for her signature.

BALANCE FORWARD			Inner City Health Care		2417
2417			222 S. First Avenue		
DATE _____ 20 ____			Carlton, MI 11666		
TO _____			(814) 555-7155		_____ 20 ___
FOR _____			PAY TO THE ORDER OF _____	$ _____	
					DOLLARS
TOTAL			First Bank		
THIS PAYMENT			5411 Brown Rd.		
BALANCE			Carlton, MI 11666		
TAX DEDUCTIBLE ☑			FOR _____ ⑆22014932		_____

Figure 17-1

C. What are five rules to ensure that checks are properly written and recorded?

(1) _____

(2) _____

(3) _____

(4) _____

(5) _____

3. A. The first rule of purchasing: Nothing is ordered or paid for without a purchase order or purchase order number. Give three reasons why it is important to ensure proper control over purchasing supplies and equipment.

(1) _____

(2) _____

(3) _____

B. Office manager Walter Seals, CMA, is responsible for purchasing office supplies for Inner City Health Care. On September 10, Walter completes purchase order #1743 for supplies ordered from Mayflower Supply, requested by administrative medical assistant Karen Ritter. The items are taxed at 8%, and the shipping fee is prepaid. The items are billed and shipped to Inner City Health Care; the terms are net due 30 days. Complete the purchase order form (Figure 17-2).

Inner City Health Care
222 S. First Avenue
Carlton, MI 11666
(814) 555-7155

Mayflower Supply, Inc.
642 East 65th Street
Carlton, MI 11623
(814) 555-9999

2 boxes of fax paper, #62145, at $8.99 a box
5 day-view desk calendars, #24598, at $4.25 each
4 cases of copier paper, #72148, at $20.00 a box
5 boxes of highlighter pens, 12 to a box, #26773, at $3.98 a box
4 computer printer cartridges, #96187, at $49.99 each

C. When the office supplies ordered from Mayflower Supply arrive, what should be done to verify that the correct items and quantities have been received? What should be done to prepare the invoice from Mayflower Supply for payment?

_____

_____

_____

_____

_____

_____

4. Describe the following types of checks, which are different from checks issued from a standard business checking account.

(1) Cashier's check _____

_____

PURCHASE ORDER

NO. 1742

Bill To:	Ship To:	Vendor:

REQ BY	BUYER	TERMS

QTY	ITEM	UNITS	DESCRIPTION	UNIT PR	TOTAL
				SUBTOTAL	
				TAX	
				FREIGHT	
				BAL DUE	

Figure 17-2

(2) Certified check _____

_____

(3) Money order _____

_____

(4) Voucher check_____

_____

(5) Traveler's check_____

5. Adjustments are entries made to a patient's account that do not represent charges or payments. Name three reasons why adjustments may sometimes be made to a patient's account.

(1) _____

(2) _____

(3) _____

6. Examine the sample bank statement in Figure 17-3; then answer the following questions.

_____ A. How many checks are not listed on the bank statement?

_____ B. What is the total amount of these outstanding checks?

_____ C. According to the bank statement, when was the last deposit made?

_____ D. What was the amount of the last deposit?

_____ E. According to Figure 17-3, what is the total of the deposits not listed on the bank statement?

_____ F. What fees did the bank charge this month?

Summary of Account Balance				Closing Date 1/15/20XX	
Account # 1257-164013				Ending Balance $8,347.62	
Beginning Balance		$7,152.18			
Total Deposits and Additions		$8,643.86			
Total Withdrawals		$7,433.21			
Service Charge		$ 15.24			
Number	Date	Amount	Number	Date	Amount
201	12/18/XX	173.82	234	1/4/XX	96.31
223*	12/18/XX	44.12	235	1/4/XX	73.48
224	12/20/XX	586.00	236	1/6/XX	325.40
225	12/21/XX	24.15	237	1/7/XX	40.00
226	12/22/XX	33.90	238	1/8/XX	66.77
228*	12/23/XX	1250.00	241*	1/9/XX	15.55
229	12/24/XX	11.75	242	1/10/XX	12.45
230	12/24/XX	19.02	243	1/10/XX	4441.25
231	1/2/XX	43.80	244	1/10/XX	64.55
232	1/3/XX	39.00			
233	1/4/XX	71.50			

*Denotes gap in check sequence

Date	Deposit Amount	Date	Deposit Amount
18-Dec	361.25	4-Jan	825.00
19-Dec	586.00	5-Jan	1286.71
20-Dec	918.21	7-Jan	608.00
21-Dec	201.00	8-Jan	811.15
2-Jan	475.00	9-Jan	1092.68
3-Jan	1478.36		

Front

1. Enter Ending Balance from the front of this statement
$ _8,347.62_

2. Enter deposits not shown on this statement
$ _3,162.50_

3. Subtotal (add 1 & 2)
$ _11,510.12_

4. List outstanding checks or other withdrawals here

Check #	Amount
222	37.89
227	161.15
239	11.50
240	92.12
245	835.17
246	21.75
247	586.00

5. Total outstanding checks
$ _1,745.58_

Balance (subtract #5 from #3)
$ _9,764.54_
This should equal your checkbook balance

Back

Figure 17-3

7. A. Deposits are generally made daily. All checks to be deposited must be endorsed. Define *endorsement*. Identify the best method of endorsing checks in the ambulatory care setting and describe the benefits of using this method.

_____

_____

_____

B. Checks received from patients and others must be inspected before preparing the checks for deposit. What guidelines should medical assistants follow in accepting and inspecting checks?

_____

_____

C. If a check is returned to the ambulatory care setting for insufficient funds, what procedures should be followed?

_____

_____

8. It is crucial to balance all financial information for each day and for the month's end. Month-end figures on the day sheet must agree with the patient ledgers. Why is it important to go through this time-consuming accounting process?

_____

_____

_____

9. A physician's fee profile is:
   a. based on an average of all the practice's fees
   b. a continuous record of usual charges made for specific services
   c. an average of fees charged over a period of 3 months
   d. is the amount paid by insurance carriers

10. A patient encounter form:
    a. might be called a charge slip
    b. used to be called a superbill
    c. is only used in computerized systems
    d. both a and b

11. The petty cash fund is kept on hand to:
    a. make change for a patient using a large bill to pay for services
    b. make funds available for all office personnel
    c. pay for minor and incidental expenses
    d. provide funds for weekly lunches for all employees

12. When a check must be guaranteed for the amount in which it is written, a _____ is issued.
    a. cashier's check
    b. certified check
    c. voucher check
    d. traveler's check

13. Restricting the use of a check should it be lost or stolen may be done through:
    a. reconciling
    b. balancing
    c. special endorsement
    d. blank endorsement

CERTIFICATION REVIEW

These questions are designed to mimic the certification examinations. You can use these questions like a small "Certification Examination Study Guide," but this is not meant to take the place of the more extensive study guides. Use this portion to determine in what areas to concentrate your efforts when studying for the certification examination.

1. The pegboard system of bookkeeping is sometimes called:
   a. the write-it-once system
   b. the ledger system
   c. the double-entry system
   d. the duplicated page system

2. NSF stands for:
   a. nonsufficient funds
   b. not sufficient funds
   c. not satisfactory funding
   d. negligent status of funding

3. A restrictive endorsement stamp is used to:
   a. stamp on the ledger to signify payment has been made
   b. stamp the doctor's signature to insurance forms and other documents
   c. stamp on the statement to signify you have sent a check
   d. stamp on the back of a check to signify "for deposit only"

4. When reconciling a bank statement:
   a. The reconciling should be done every month.
   b. The checkbook entries should be checked against the bank statement.
   c. The reconciling should be done daily by computer.
   d. All reconciling should be done in ink to avoid any unauthorized entries.
   e. a and b

CASE STUDY

Suzanne Berry is a new patient at the offices of Drs. Lewis and King in the Inner City Health Care. Suzanne is a single mother of two small children. Suzanne and her children are covered by medical insurance through her employer. The policy covers 80% of the usual, reasonable, and customary fees for the family's medical expenses after a $100 per person deductible, which the Berrys have already reached from expenses incurred with the family's previous health care provider. Inner City Health Care requires that patients pay for services not covered by insurance at the time of treatment. The office also charges for all scheduled office visits, unless the patient provides a 24-hour notice of cancellation. The practice accepts personal checks, major credit cards, and, under special circumstances, installment payments.

Discuss the following:

1. Take the role of office manager Marilyn Johnson, who meets with Suzanne during her first office visit, and explain the practice's policies regarding patient fees and financial obligations.
2. Suzanne asks Marilyn to clarify what she means by "usual, reasonable, and customary fees." Explain.
3. Suzanne tells Marilyn she is interested in the option of charging some larger medical fees to her credit card. What should Marilyn explain to Suzanne about the use of credit cards in the ambulatory care setting?

SELF-ASSESSMENT

1. In your personal checkbook or banking system at home, how often do you reconcile?

2. When you do reconcile, do you balance? How much time will you spend on the reconciliation to balance?

If you reconcile your bank statements on a regular basis and balance each month, congratulations! If you do not reconcile on a regular basis, start today. Gather your last bank statement. If you do not have one, call the bank and have them send you one or download one from the Internet if your bank offers Internet banking. Accept the beginning balance on the bank statement. Gather the check stubs/copies that you have written within the bank statement beginning and end dates. Check off all the checks that have gone through the bank and are listed on the statement. Add up the outstanding checks (i.e., the ones that have not gone through yet). Subtract them from the ending balance. Add in any interest you have earned for the month. Subtract any fees you have been charged. Does your amount match the bank statement? If not, go back over your math to make sure you added and subtracted correctly and fix any errors. If you still cannot balance, call the bank and ask to sit down with a representative/clerk so they can help you balance. After you balance once, the next month will be much easier.

If your bank offers Internet or online banking, and you are not using that option, consider it. Why are you not using it? Talk to a representative to be sure the online service is secure and your information is protected. If you are satisfied that it is a safe and secure service, consider taking advantage of the online option. Reconciling the monthly statements online is easy to do because the math is done for you by the computer! If you are using online banking, do you think it saves you time? Does it save you money? Is it easier than reconciling manually?

CHAPTER POST-TEST

This is similar to the Pre-Test. Perform this test without looking at the book. This is just to see how well you have understood and can recall the information presented in this chapter after you have studied it and completed the workbook exercises. You will not be graded on this portion (other than the grade you give yourself), but this is an excellent preparation for your instructor's test. You may use this Post-Test to determine what areas you need to study more. Justify any "false" answers.

1. The management of the business details is often the responsibility of the medical assisting staff. (T or F)

2. The same fees for services should be charged to every patient, regardless of whether they have insurance coverage. (T or F)

3. You should encourage the use of credit/debit cards for medical bills. (T or F)

4. Purchase orders are to be written up before the purchase is made. (T or F)

5. Petty cash is available for authorized use when the employees need cash. (T or F)

CERTIFICATION CRITERIA CHECKLIST

As you go through your education and training, keep in mind the national certification examination that you will take when you graduate. Each chapter of the textbook and workbook covers a different section of the examination criteria. To keep track of your preparation for the certification examination, turn to the back of this workbook and highlight the following CMA, RMA, or CMAS certification examination criteria (if you have already highlighted them from a previous chapter, put a check mark by the criteria):

CMA
O.   Managing the Office
      2.   Equipment and supply inventory
Q.   Managing Practice Finances
      1.   Bookkeeping systems
      4.   Accounting and banking procedures

RMA
II.   Administrative Medical Assisting
      B.   Finance/Bookkeeping

CMAS
1.   Medical Office Financial Management
      •   Fundamental financial management
      •   Patient accounts
      •   Banking

COMPETENCY ASSESSMENT
Procedure 17-1 Recording/Posting Patient Charges, Payments, and Adjustments

Performance Objectives: To record information including services rendered, fees charged, any adjustments made, and balances pertaining to a patient's visit to the physician and the patient's account. Perform this objective within 15 minutes with a minimum score of 55 points.

Supplies/Equipment: Calculator, computer, patient's account or ledger

Charting/Documentation: Enter appropriate documentation/charting in the box.

_____

_____

_____

_____

Instructor's/Evaluator's Comments and Suggestions:

_____

_____

_____

_____

_____

SKILLS CHECKLIST Procedure 17-1: Recording/Posting Patient Charges, Payments, and Adjustments

Name _____

Date _____

No.	Skill	Check #1 20 pts ea	Check #2 10 pts ea	Check #3 5 pts ea	Notes
1	Check patient's account before appointment to ensure it is up to date.				
2	When patient arrives, check for name, address, telephone number, and any changes in medical insurance.				
3	Fill encounter form or superbill, and attach to the patient's medical chart.				
4	When the physician completes the examination, he or she will check the procedures and diagnosis on the encounter form.				
5	Read the encounter form and calculate the total cost for procedures.				
6	Post each service as a charge or debit. Post payments received as a credit.				
7	Apply any adjustments.				
8	Determine the current balance.				
9	If recording a payment, place a restrictive endorsement on the check.				
10	Record the payment.				
11	Place cash or processed check in the appointed place.				
Student's Total Points					
Points Possible		220	110	55	
Final Score (Student's Total Points / Possible Points)					

	Notes
Start time:	
End time:	
Total time: (15 min goal)	

COMPETENCY ASSESSMENT
Procedure 17-2 Balancing Day Sheets in a Manual System

Performance Objectives: To verify that all entries to the day sheet are correct and that the totals balance. Perform this objective within 15 minutes with a minimum score of 55 points.

Supplies/Equipment: Day sheet, calculator

Charting/Documentation: Enter appropriate documentation/charting in the box.

_____

_____

_____

_____

Instructor's/Evaluator's Comments and Suggestions:

_____

_____

_____

_____

_____

_____

SKILLS CHECKLIST Procedure 17-2: Balancing Day Sheets in a Manual System

Name _____

Date _____

No.	Skill	Check #1 20 pts ea	Check #2 10 pts ea	Check #3 5 pts ea	Notes
1	Total columns A, B1, B2, C, and D.				
2	Proof of posting: verify that $D + A - B = C$.				
3	Fill encounter form or superbill, and attach to the patient's medical chart.				
4	When the physician completes the examination, he or she will check the procedures and diagnosis on the encounter form.				
5	Read the encounter form, and calculate the total cost for procedures.				
6	Post each service as a charge or debit. Post payments received as a credit.				
7	Apply any adjustments.				
8	Determine the current balance.				
9	If recording a payment, place a restrictive endorsement on the check.				
10	Record the payment.				
11	Place cash or processed check in the appointed place.				
Student's Total Points					
Points Possible		220	110	55	
Final Score (Student's Total Points / Possible Points)					

	Notes
Start time:	
End time:	
Total time: (15 min goal)	

COMPETENCY ASSESSMENT
Procedure 17-3 Preparing a Deposit

Performance Objectives: To create a deposit slip for the day's receipts. Perform this objective within 15 minutes with a minimum score of 50 points.

Supplies/Equipment: New deposit slip, check endorsement stamp, calculator, cash and checks received for the day

Charting/Documentation: Enter appropriate documentation/charting in the box.

_____

_____

_____

_____

Instructor's/Evaluator's Comments and Suggestions:

_____

_____

_____

_____

_____

_____

SKILLS CHECKLIST Procedure 17-3: Preparing a Deposit

Name _____

Date _____

No.	Skill	Check #1 20 pts ea	Check #2 10 pts ea	Check #3 5 pts ea	Notes
1	Separate checks from currency.				
2	Count currency and enter amount in space provided. Gather bills in order, facing the same direction.				
3	Count all coins, and enter amount in space provided.				
4	On the back of the deposit slip, list each check separately. Include patient's name and amount of check.				
5	Total the checks listed and copy the total on the front.				
6	Verify that sum of currency, coins, and checks equals the total payments on day sheet.				
7	Attach top copy of deposit slip to deposit.				
8	Enter date and amount of the deposit on checkbook stubs.				
9	Add the amount of deposit to the checkbook balance.				
10	Deposit at the bank.				
Student's Total Points					
Points Possible		200	100	50	
Final Score (Student's Total Points / Possible Points)					

	Notes
Start time:	
End time:	
Total time: (15 min goal)	

COMPETENCY ASSESSMENT

Procedure 17-4 Reconciling a Bank Statement

Performance Objectives: To verify that the balance listed in the checkbook agrees with the balance shown by the bank. Perform this objective within 15 minutes with a minimum score of 55 points.

Supplies/Equipment: Checkbook, bank statement, calculator

Charting/Documentation: Enter appropriate documentation/charting in the box.

_____

_____

_____

_____

Instructor's/Evaluator's Comments and Suggestions:

_____

_____

_____

_____

_____

SKILLS CHECKLIST Procedure 17-4: Reconciling a Bank Statement

Name _____

Date _____

No.	Skill	Check #1 20 pts ea	Check #2 10 pts ea	Check #3 5 pts ea	Notes
1	Make sure the balance in the checkbook is current.				
2	Subtract any service charge listed from the last balance in the checkbook.				
3	In the checkbook, check off each check listed on the statement and verify the amount against the check stub.				
4	In the checkbook, check off each deposit listed on the statement.				
5	The back of the statement contains a worksheet for balancing.				
6	Copy the ending balance from the front of the statement to the back.				
7	Go through the check stubs and record on the back of the statement any checks that have not cleared, or deposits that were not shown as received.				
8	Total the checks not cleared on the statement worksheet.				
9	Total the deposits not credited on the worksheet.				
10	Add together the statement balance and the total of deposits not credited.				
11	Subtract the total of checks not cleared. Verify with the balance in the checkbook. File the statement worksheet.				
Student's Total Points					
Points Possible		220	110	55	
Final Score (Student's Total Points / Possible Points)					

	Notes
Start time:	
End time:	
Total time: (15 min goal)	

COMPETENCY ASSESSMENT

Procedure 17-5 Balancing Petty Cash

Performance Objectives: To verify that the amount of petty cash is consistent with the beginning amount less expenditures shown on receipts. Perform this objective within 15 minutes with a minimum score of 45 points.

Supplies/Equipment: Petty cash box with cash balance, vouchers, calculator

Charting/Documentation: Enter appropriate documentation/charting in the box.

_____

_____

_____

_____

Instructor's/Evaluator's Comments and Suggestions:

_____

_____

_____

_____

_____

SKILLS CHECKLIST Procedure 17-5: Balancing Petty Cash

Name _____

Date _____

No.	Skill	Check #1 20 pts ea	Check #2 10 pts ea	Check #3 5 pts ea	Notes
1	Count the money in the box.				
2	Total the amount of all vouchers.				
3	Subtract the amount of receipts from the original amount.				
4	When cash has been balanced, write a check only for the amount that was used.				
Check Disbursement:					
5	Sort all vouchers by account.				
6	On a sheet of paper, list the accounts.				
7	Total vouchers for each account, then record individual totals.				
8	Copy the list totals onto the "memo" portion of the stub for the replenishment check.				
9	File the list with the vouchers and receipts attached, noting the check number.				
Student's Total Points					
Points Possible		180	90	45	
Final Score (Student's Total Points / Possible Points)					

	Notes
Start time:	
End time:	
Total time: (15 min goal)	

COMPETENCY ASSESSMENT

Procedure 17-6 Recording a Nonsufficient Funds Check

Performance Objectives: To perform bookkeeping functions that keep account in proper balance. Perform this objective within 15 minutes with a minimum score of 20 points.

Supplies/Equipment: The practice's account balance, manual day sheet or computerized practice account, manual ledger or computerized patient account, NSF check

Charting/Documentation: Enter appropriate documentation/charting in the box.

_____

_____

_____

_____

Instructor's/Evaluator's Comments and Suggestions:

_____

_____

_____

_____

_____

_____

SKILLS CHECKLIST Procedure 17-6: Recording a Nonsufficient Funds Check

Name _____

Date _____

No.	Skill	Check #1 20 pts ea	Check #2 10 pts ea	Check #3 5 pts ea	Notes
1	Follow the office policy for notifying the patient.				
2	When the NSF check has been returned the second time, deduct the check amount from the account balance of the practice.				
3	Add the amount of the NSF check back into the patient's account or ledger.				
4	Place a brief explanation in the description column.				
Student's Total Points					
Points Possible		80	40	20	
Final Score (Student's Total Points / Possible Points)					

	Notes
Start time:	
End time:	
Total time: (15 min goal)	

EVALUATION OF CHAPTER KNOWLEDGE

Skills	Student Self-Evaluation		
	Good	Average	Poor
I can define the key vocabulary terms in this chapter.	____	____	____
I can demonstrate understanding of procedures, policies, and services.	____	____	____
I understand the importance of informing patients of the office's financial policies and procedures.	____	____	____
I can document various financial forms correctly.	____	____	____
I understand documentation and reporting needs.	____	____	____
I am able to use manual bookkeeping systems.	____	____	____
I can apply computer concepts to computerized accounting systems.	____	____	____
I can demonstrate the ability to manage accounts receivable.	____	____	____
I can demonstrate the ability to manage accounts payable.	____	____	____
I am able to establish, track, balance, and replenish a petty cash fund.	____	____	____
I can write and record checks and reconcile accounts.	____	____	____
I can demonstrate an understanding of purchasing procedures and the ability to prepare purchase orders.	____	____	____

CHAPTER 18

Medical Insurance

CHAPTER PRE-TEST

Perform this test without looking at the book. This is just to see how well you have understood and can recall the information in this chapter after you have read it, but before you have completed the workbook exercises. You will not be graded on this portion (other than the grade you give yourself). Justify any "false" answers.

1. Managed care has simplified the patient's responsibility for payment. (T or F)
2. With managed care options, there is less emphasis on the medical assistant needing to be accurate and timely when filing insurance claims. (T or F)
3. Preexisting conditions usually require a waiting period. (T or F)
4. Coordination of benefits means that the insurance companies will take care of the paperwork. (T or F)
5. Copayment is the amount the insurance will cost the patient each month. (T or F)

INTRODUCTION

With the growing influence of managed care, many traditional insurance carriers, such as Blue Cross and Blue Shield, are joining health maintenance organizations (HMOs) and other managed care options in transforming the health care insurance industry. Students also discover the medical assistant's important role as a patient educator, helping patients understand the terms and conditions of their health insurance policies.

PERFORMANCE OBJECTIVES

After successful completion of this chapter you will be able to explain the terminology related to medical insurances. You will be able to recall several different examples of medical insurance coverage and discuss their similarities and differences. You will be familiar with several primary managed care organization models and recall the steps involved when screening patients for insurance coverage. You will know about legal and ethical issues related to medical insurance and the physician's office, including the impacts of Health Insurance Portability and Accountability Act (HIPAA) requirements. You will also be aware of the importance of obtaining referrals and preauthorizations from insurance companies before providing services and the ramifications if the referrals or preauthorizations are overlooked. *The following statements are related to your learning objectives from this chapter. Fill in the blanks in the following paragraph with the appropriate term(s).*

The term used to describe the person who is insured is (1) _____. The amount of money that the insured person must incur before the insurance policy begins to pay is called the (2) _____. Some insurance policies require that the patient pay a certain amount at the time of service. This is called the (3) _____.

A disease or disorder the patient has before he or she opens his or her insurance policy may not be covered for a certain amount of time, because it is considered to be a (4) _____ _____ condition. Sometimes insurance policies will not cover procedures and treatments either because they are considered not to be medically necessary or perhaps they have not been proved to be effective. These procedures or treatments are called (5) _____. Before some services are allowed, they must first be approved by the insurance company. The process for getting this approval is called (6) _____ _____. Many traditional insurance policies require patients to choose one physician who will coordinate all their care. This physician is known as their PCP. PCP is an abbreviation for (7) _____. Some policies even limit the physicians from whom patients can seek treatment. The patients must choose their specialists from a list of approved physicians who have contracted with the insurance company. These physicians are considered to be (8) _____. A list of approved medications can be found on the (9) _____.

If a medication is not on the list, the patient will have to pay more for it. Fee schedules are determined from a variety of elements, including the (10) _____ or practice expenses, the cost of (11) _____, and the (12) _____ for the services provided by the physician. All of these cost elements combined with the (13) _____ required is used to determine a fee schedule. UCR, or (14) _____ _____ Fee Schedule defines the allowable fees accepted by insurance carriers. Medicare has a system called RBRVS, or (15) _____ _____, in which physician's services are reimbursed based on relative value. This formula takes into consideration not only the physician's overhead expenses, the work involved, and malpractice expenses, but also a (16) _____ practice cost index. (17) _____ _____ is a payment system used by managed care organizations in which a fixed dollar amount is reimbursed to the physician. This type of system requires the physician to practice extensive (18) _____ to be effective. HIPAA stands for (19) _____

and includes several rules. One of the rules, HIPAA privacy requirements, addresses issues of

(20) _____. These rules state that the practice must

provide the patient with a (21) _____ form

that outlines the provider's privacy practices. Another requirement is that the practice obtain

(22) _____ from the patient to use or disclose per-

sonal information. The practice must also provide the patient, on request, an accounting of any

(23) _____ of protected information.

VOCABULARY BUILDER

Find the words below that are misspelled; circle them, and then correctly spell them in the spaces provided. Then insert the correct vocabulary terms from the list that best fit the descriptions below.

point of service plan	referral
preautherization	resourse-based relative value scale
prefered provider organization	self-insurance
primary care physician/provider	usual, customary, and reasonible
proof of eligibility	Worker's Compensation insurance

_____   _____

_____   _____

_____

1. The _____ is a doctor chosen
   by the patient who is the first doctor the patient sees and is responsible for making referrals
   for further treatment by a specialist or for hospitalization.

2. A _____ allows the enrollee to
   have the freedom to obtain medical care from an HMO provider or to self-refer to a non-
   HMO provider at a greater cost.

3. In a _____, enrollees obtain ser-
   vices from a network of physicians and hospitals who have contracted with the insurance
   company.

4. _____ was devel-
   oped using values for each medical and surgical procedure based on work, practice, and
   malpractice costs and factoring in the regional differences.

5. _____ requirement means that prior notice and
   approval needs to be obtained before services will be covered.

LEARNING REVIEW

1. What questions should the medical assistant ask when screening for medical insurance coverage?

   A. _____

   B. _____

   C. _____

   D. _____

2. List five measures that managed care organizations (MCOs) employ to ensure cost-effective services.

   A. _____

   B. _____

   C. _____

   D. _____

   E. _____

3. What are the six MCO models in use?

   A. _____

   B. _____

   C. _____

   D. _____

   E. _____

   F. _____

4. List seven pieces of information that should be maintained in a log regarding preauthorization, precertification, or referral procedures for various insurance carriers.

   A. _____

   B. _____

   C. _____

   D. _____

   E. _____

   F. _____

   G. _____

5. Identify the three common elements involved in computing a physician's fee schedule.

   A. _____

   B. _____

   C. _____

6. Which of the following is a problem with work-related health insurance coverage?
   a. part-time employees are not usually eligible
   b. medical benefits may not transfer equally
   c. insurance companies often refuse to provide coverage for some procedures, including experimental treatments
   d. all of the above

7. The person covered under the terms of an insurance policy is called the:
   a. primary
   b. secondary
   c. beneficiary
   d. elector

8. When more than one policy covers the individual, the _____ determines which of the policies will pay first.
   a. deductible
   b. exclusion
   c. coinsurance
   d. coordination of benefits

9. Where does one find the address to which insurance claims are to be sent?
   a. the telephone book
   b. on the back of the insurance card
   c. in the insurance provider manual
   d. none of the above

10. Blue Cross and Blue Shield are examples of a:
    a. managed care organization (MCO)
    b. health maintenance organization (HMO)
    c. preferred provider organization (PPO)
    d. traditional insurance organization

CERTIFICATION REVIEW

These questions are designed to mimic the certification examinations. You can use these questions like a small "Certification Examination Study Guide," but this is not meant to take the place of the more extensive study guides. Use this portion to determine in what areas to concentrate your efforts when studying for the certification examination. Justify any "false" answers.

1. The portion of the medical fees that the patient needs to pay at the time of services is called a:
   a. copay
   b. fee for service
   c. out of pocket expenses
   d. premium

2. The cost patients must pay each month (sometimes provided by their employers) is called the:

   a. out of pocket expenses

   b. copay

   c. premium

   d. relative value scale

3. HIPAA:

   a. is about confidentiality, patient privacy, and security of personal health information

   b. protects health insurance coverage for workers and their families when they change or lose their jobs

   c. includes national standards for electronic health care transactions

   d. establishes rules for national identifiers for providers, health plans, and employers

   e. all of the above

4. Electronic medical records have made confidentiality easier to protect. (T or F)

CASE STUDY

Lourdes Austen, a one-year survivor of breast cancer, is covered by an HMO. Lourdes's primary care physician, Dr. King, recommends that Lourdes receive a colonoscopy because she has a family history that is positive for colon cancer; medical studies have demonstrated a link between colon and breast cancers in families. Lourdes's HMO requires preauthorization before a specialist's care can be provided. Dr. King supplies the referral to a gastroenterologist who will perform the colon screening test and gives Lourdes the necessary completed referral form to take with her to her scheduled appointment.

During the colonoscopy procedure, one benign polyp is removed, and the gastroenterologist requests that Lourdes return for a follow-up examination in one week. Lourdes makes an appointment with the specialist's administrative medical assistant. When she returns one week later, the medical assistant informs Lourdes that she must have a new referral form for the office visit or the HMO will not approve payment; Lourdes will have to pay for the examination herself. "But we drove 40 minutes to get here, and no one ever told me I'd need another form for this. I thought it was all covered under the colonoscopy," Lourdes says.

Discuss the following:

1. Lourdes's HMO policy requires preauthorization. Is there anything that can be done to secure a proper referral without having to schedule another appointment for the patient or force the patient to pay for the office visit?

2. What is the role of the specialist's administrative medical assistant in this situation? Could the situation have been prevented?

SELF-ASSESSMENT

1. Take a close look at your insurance coverage. If you do not have medical insurance coverage, take a look at the coverage of a close friend or relative or choose a policy you would like to have.

   A. Does it require a copay?

   B. How much is the copay for a doctor's visit?

   C. How much is the copay for a hospital stay? Surgery?

   D. How much is the copay for medication?

   E. Does prescribed medication have to be from a formulary list?

   F. How much is the total amount you would have to pay for any given year?

2. Some people advocate doing away with health insurance for office visits and medications and just having insurance for big expenses such as catastrophic coverage. Discuss this idea with a group of at least three people. These people may be your classmates or friends/family. Write up a list of the advantages and disadvantages.

3. Some people advocate a "socialistic" method of health insurance such as Canada has. Look online for information about Canada's health care system and make a list of the advantages and disadvantages. Which way would you vote if you had a choice?

CHAPTER POST-TEST

This is similar to the Pre-Test. Perform this test without looking at the book. This is just to see how well you have understood and can recall the information presented in this chapter after you have studied it and completed the workbook exercises. You will not be graded on this portion (other than the grade you give yourself), but this is an excellent preparation for your instructor's test. You may use this Post-Test to determine what areas you need to study more. Justify any "false" answers.

1. Managed care has made the patient's responsibility for payment more complex. (T or F)

2. With managed care options, there is more emphasis on the medical assistant needing to be accurate and timely when filing insurance claims. (T or F)

3. Preexisting conditions always require a waiting period. (T or F)

4. Coordination of benefits means that the insurance companies will handle all the paperwork necessary for payment. (T or F)

5. Copayment is the amount the insurance will cost the patient's employer each month. (T or F)

CERTIFICATION CRITERIA CHECKLIST

As you go through your education and training, keep in mind the national certification examination that you will take when you graduate. Each chapter of the textbook and workbook covers a different section of the examination criteria. To keep track of your preparation for the certification examination, turn to the back of this workbook and highlight the following CMA, RMA, or CMAS certification examination criteria (if you have already highlighted them from a previous chapter, put a check mark by the criteria):

CMA
F.   Medicolegal Guidelines & Requirements
    2.   Legislation
    5.   Physician-patient relationship
Q.   Managing Practice Finances
    3.   Third-party billing

RMA
II.   Administrative Medical Assisting
    A.   Insurance

CMAS
5.   Health Care Insurance Processing, Coding and Billing
- Insurance processing
- Insurance billing and finances

COMPETENCY ASSESSMENT

Procedure 18-1 Screening for Insurance

Performance Objectives: To verify insurance coverage and obtain vital information required for processing and billing insurance claim forms. Perform this objective within 15 minutes with a minimum score of 25 points.

Supplies/Equipment: Patient registration forms, clipboard and black ink pen, patient's chart

Charting/Documentation: Enter appropriate documentation/charting in the box.

_____

_____

_____

_____

Instructor's/Evaluator's Comments and Suggestions:

_____

_____

_____

_____

_____

SKILLS CHECKLIST Procedure 18-1: Screening for Insurance

Name _____

Date _____

No.	Skill	Check #1 20 pts ea	Check #2 10 pts ea	Check #3 5 pts ea	Notes
1	Ask patients to bring their insurance cards, and arrive 15–20 minutes before appointment time.				
2	Review completed patient registration form for legibility and completeness.				
3	Make front and back photocopies of patient's insurance card and attach to patient's chart.				
4	Verify proof of eligibility for Medicaid patients.				
5	Each time patient checks in, verify address and insurance coverage. Check insurance card. Determine that their primary care physician is performing the procedure and that the procedure is covered.				
Student's Total Points					
Points Possible		100	50	25	
Final Score (Student's Total Points / Possible Points)					

	Notes
Start time:	
End time:	
Total time: (15 min goal)	

COMPETENCY ASSESSMENT

Procedure 18-2 Obtaining Referrals and Authorizations

Performance Objectives: To ascertain coverage by the insurance carrier for specific medical services, hospital admissions, inpatient or outpatient surgeries, elective procedures, or when the primary care physician elects to refer the patient to another physician. Perform this objective within 15 minutes with a minimum score of 35 points.

Supplies/Equipment: Patient's medical chart and copy of the patient's insurance card, name of the carrier contact person and telephone number, completed referral form, telephone/fax machine, pen/pencil

Charting/Documentation: Enter appropriate documentation/charting in the box.

Instructor's/Evaluator's Comments and Suggestions:

SKILLS CHECKLIST Procedure 18-2: Obtaining Referrals and Authorizations

Name _____

Date _____

No.	Skill	Check #1 20 pts ea	Check #2 10 pts ea	Check #3 5 pts ea	Notes
1	Collect all necessary documents and equipment.				
2	Determine the service or procedure requiring preauthorization.				
3	Complete the referral form.				
4	Proofread the completed form.				
5	Fax the completed form to the insurance carrier.				
6	Maintain a completed copy of the referral form in the patient's chart.				
7	Maintain a completed copy of the authorization number/ code in the patient's chart.				
Student's Total Points					
Points Possible		140	70	35	
Final Score (Student's Total Points / Possible Points)					

	Notes
Start time:	
End time:	
Total time: (15 min goal)	

EVALUATION OF CHAPTER KNOWLEDGE

Skills	Student Self-Evaluation		
	Good	Average	Poor
I can describe the history of medical insurance in this country and its evolution in recent years.	———	———	———
I can define the terminology necessary to understand and submit medical insurance claims.	———	———	———
I know at least five examples of medical insurance coverage.	———	———	———
I can explain the significance of diagnosis-related groups.	———	———	———
I am comfortable as a patient educator about insurance issues.	———	———	———

CHAPTER 19

Medical Insurance Coding

CHAPTER PRE-TEST

Perform this test without looking at the book. This is just to see how well you have understood and can recall the information in this chapter after you have read it, but before you have completed the workbook exercises. You will not be graded on this portion (other than the grade you give yourself). Justify any "false" answers.

1. Medical insurance coding is a way of keeping track of the doctor's financial records. (T or F)

2. CPT stands for:
   a. Comprehensive Patient Treatments
   b. Current Procedural Terminology
   c. Curative Procedures Tried
   d. Curative Patient Treatments

3. ICD stands for:
   a. Incidental Codes of Diagnosis
   b. Internal Codes for Decisions
   c. International Codes for Diagnosis
   d. International Classifications of Diseases

4. Third party usually means the insurance company. (T or F)

5. Insurance claim forms and submissions are fairly straightforward; therefore, most anyone can perform these duties with some basic training. (T or F)

INTRODUCTION

Although managed care coverage has simplified the patient's responsibility for payment in some ways, medical assistants have the responsibility to be accurate, timely, and conscientious both in filing insurance claim forms and in understanding the conditions of individual insurance policies. Medical assisting students can use this workbook chapter to explore the role of insurance, learn insurance terminology, and apply accurate insurance coding of diagnosis and procedure codes.

PERFORMANCE OBJECTIVES

After successful completion of this chapter you will be able to explain the terminology related to medical insurance coding. You will understand the process of procedure and diagnostic coding and will be able to code a simple claim form. You will be able to explain the difference between the Centers for Medicare and Medicaid Services Form 1500 (CMS-1500) and the Uniform Bill 92 (UB92) forms, and discuss why claims follow-up is important. You will also be able to discuss legal and ethical issues related to medical coding and insurance claims processing. *The following statements are related to your learning objectives from this chapter. Fill in the blanks in the following paragraph with the appropriate term(s).*

The advent of computers has required that diagnoses and procedures be put into (1) _____ format. The CPT system was developed by the (2) _____ to convert descriptions of procedures into numbers. The (3) _____ developed the ICD-9 CM to classify diseases in the same way. The current ICD-9 CM codes consist of (4) _____ digit codes with (5) _____ modifiers. (6) _____ is a way for insurance companies to reduce the reimbursement amounts if the documentation or codes are ambiguous. There are three ways this can happen: (7) _____, (8) _____, or (9) _____. Up coding, also known as (10) _____, (11) _____, or (12) _____, occurs when the insurance carrier is deliberately billed at a higher rate service than was performed to obtain a greater reimbursement. The CPT is divided into (13) _____ sections. One of the sections, called the (14) _____ section, takes every possible combination of visits into consideration and assigns each its own number. Occasionally, a service or procedure needs to be modified, so there is an optional two-digit numeric (15) _____ that can be applied as an explanation. Medicare created the (16) _____ _____ system for their patients. This system has three levels. Level I uses the basic system. Level II provides codes for (17) _____

_____, (18) _____, and

(19) _____. Level III codes are defined by Medi-

care regional (20) _____ carriers.

VOCABULARY BUILDER

A. *Find the words below that are misspelled; circle them, and then correctly spell them in the spaces provided.*

bindled codes	Healthcare Common Procedure Coding System
claim register	insurance abuse
Current Procedural Terminoligy	International Classification of Deseases
E Codes	point-of-service device
encounter form	U Codes
explanation of benifits	Uniform Bill
fraud	

_____   _____

_____   _____

B. *Write the definition of the following terms or phrases.*

1. Bundled codes

_____

2. Claim register

_____

3. *Current Procedural Terminology (CPT)*

_____

4. E Codes

_____

5. Encounter form

_____

6. Explanation of Benefits (EOB)

_____

7. Fraud

_____

8. Healthcare Common Procedure Coding System (HCPCS)

_____

9. Insurance abuse

_____

10. International Classification of Diseases, 9th Revision, Clinical Modifications (ICD-9-CM)

_____

11. Point-of-service (POS) device

_____

12. Uniform Bill (UB92)

_____

13. V Codes

_____

LEARNING REVIEW

1. Coding for procedures done and for visits of all kinds—office, hospital, nursing facility, home services—is found in *CPT*.

   A. *CPT* is divided into seven sections. This volume is updated annually and published by the American Medical Association. Name the seven sections.

   (1) _____   (5) _____

   (2) _____   (6) _____

   (3) _____   (7) _____

   (4) _____

   B. For each procedure listed, give the correct procedure code and name the *CPT* section in which the code can be found.

   1. Chemotherapy administration, infusion technique, up to 1 hour

      code: _____   section: _____

   2. Hepatitis B surface antibody

      code: _____   section: _____

   3. Simple repair of superficial wounds of scalp, neck, axillae, external genitalia, trunk or extremities (including hands and feet) 7.6 to 12.5 cm

      code: _____   section: _____

   4. Electrocardiogram, routine ECG with 12 leads; with interpretation and reports

      code: _____   section: _____

5. Hepatic venography, wedged or free, with hemodynamic evaluation, radiologic supervision, and interpretation

code: _____   section: _____

6. Hepatitis Be antigen (HBeAg)

code: _____   section: _____

7. Anesthesia for arthroscopic procedures of hip joint

code: _____   section: _____

2. A. Codes for diagnoses are found in the ICD-9-CM. ICD-9-CM is divided into three volumes. Specify below what information each volume contains.

Volume I: _____

_____

Volume II: _____

_____

Volume III: _____

_____

B. Provide answers to the following questions:

In which volume of the ICD would a medical assistant first look to find the diagnosis code for osteomyelitis? (1) _____ What is the diagnosis code for unspecified osteomyelitis of the ankle or foot? (2) _____ Injury codes cannot stand alone, but must be accompanied by "E" Codes. What do E Codes stand for? (3) _____ What is the diagnosis code for obesity? (4) _____ "V" Codes are the last main section of Volumes I and II. What do V Codes stand for? (5) _____

_____.

3. Errors in coding insurance claims can have far-reaching effects for both the patient and the physician. Name three effects.

(1) _____

_____

(2) _____

_____

(3) _____

_____

4. For each entry in the following table, insert a "D" for diagnosis or "P" for procedure on the first line. Then, enter the appropriate diagnosis or procedure code, referencing this textbook, the current revision of the ICD, or the current edition of the CPT. In the explanation column, identify whether the procedures are laboratory procedures (LAB), part of the physician's physical examination process (PE), diagnostic procedures (DP), examples of medication administration (MA), preventive measures (PM), procedures related to litigation (LEG), or rehabilitative medicine procedures (RP). For each diagnosis, give a brief definition of the patient condition or illness, consulting a medical encyclopedia if necessary.

Diagnosis/ Procedure	Entry	Code	Explanation
_____	1. Services requested after hours in addition to basic services	_____	_____
_____	2. Medicine given or taken in error	_____	_____
_____	3. Anorexia nervosa	_____	_____
_____	4. Pneumonocentesis, puncture of lung for aspiration	_____	_____
_____	5. Diabetic ketoacidosis	_____	_____
_____	6. Urinalysis; qualitative or semi-quantitative, except immunoassays, microscopic only	_____	_____
_____	7. Bruxism	_____	_____
_____	8. *Pneumocystis carinii* pneumonia	_____	_____
_____	9. Amniocentesis	_____	_____
_____	10. Epstein–Barr virus infection	_____	_____
_____	11. Gait training (includes stair climbing)	_____	_____
_____	12. Medical testimony	_____	_____
_____	13. DTP (diphtheria-tetanus-pertussis) vaccination	_____	_____
_____	14. Therapeutic or diagnostic injection (specify material injected); subcutaneous or intramuscular	_____	_____
_____	15. Narcotics affecting fetus via placenta or breast milk	_____	_____

5. Differentiate between bundled and unbundled codes.

_____

_____

_____

6. List five common errors committed when completing insurance claim forms.

    (1) _____

    (2) _____

    (3) _____

    (4) _____

    (5) _____

7. Identify seven basic elements necessary to have documented in a compliance program.

    (1) _____

    (2) _____

    (3) _____

    (4) _____

    (5) _____

    (6) _____

    (7) _____

8. Using the number of patients enrolled in a health maintenance organization (HMO) to determine a physician's salary is called:

    a. coinsurance

    b. capitation

    c. catchment

    d. assignment

9. Part A of Medicare covers:

    a. hospice care

    b. physical therapy

    c. diagnostic tests

    d. ambulance services

10. Using an electronic device for direct communication between medical offices and a health care plan's computer is called:

    a. subrogation

    b. point of service

    c. diagnosis-related groups

    d. prospective payment

11. The most common claim form for the ambulatory setting is the:
    a. HCFA-1500
    b. HCFA-1000
    c. CMS 1500
    d. CPT 1500

12. The codes that show a patient has been seen for reasons other than sickness or injury are:
    a. S Codes
    b. D Codes
    c. V Codes
    d. X Codes

CERTIFICATION REVIEW

These questions are designed to mimic the certification examinations. You can use these questions like a small "Certification Examination Study Guide," but this is not meant to take the place of the more extensive study guides. Use this portion to determine in what areas to concentrate your efforts when studying for the certification examination.

1. What is the name of the coding system that includes codes for services provided to Medicare or Medicaid patients?
    a. HCFA
    b. CPT
    c. ICD-9
    d. HCPCS
    e. WHO

2. If a doctor believes a claim has been denied in error, which of the following is a valid course of action he or she can take?
    a. contact the assistant attorney general
    b. begin a lawsuit
    c. begin an appeal process
    d. write off the charges
    e. bill the patient

3. A Certified Professional Coder has coded a diagnosis of 670.51. What system is he or she using?
    a. CPT
    b. ICD 9
    c. ICD 10
    d. HCPCS
    e. RVS

4. In the *CPT* manual, the description of the level of E&M codes includes which of the following?

    a. complexity of the medical decision making

    b. level of history taken

    c. number of systems examined and documented

    d. new versus established patient

    e. all of the above

5. Which of the following describes Volume II of the ICD-9?

    a. known as the Tabular Index, lists all diagnostic codes in numeric order

    b. is an alphabetical listing of diagnoses.

    c. lists procedures in tabular form

    d. all of the above

CASE STUDY

Refer to the case study presented in Chapter 18 of this workbook.

Lourdes's colonoscopy required the following diagnoses and procedures. Give the correct coding for processing the insurance claim for this patient.

colonoscopy with biopsy, single or multiple_____

flex sig (colon) _____

family history, malignant neoplasm gastrointestinal tract _____

personal history, malignant neoplasm, breast _____

low-complexity office visit _____

SELF-ASSESSMENT

A. Have you considered whether you would like to be an insurance coder and biller? Think about the following questions.

    1. What qualities do you possess that would make you a good candidate for a career in medical billing and coding?

    2. What qualities do you not possess but could obtain?

    3. What do you think you would like best about a position in medical coding and billing?

    4. What would be your least favorite part of the job?

B. Explore the profession of medical coding by looking on the Internet for coding organizations offering certification examinations. Differentiate between the various credentials available to coders.

CHAPTER POST-TEST

This is similar to the Pre-Test. Perform this test without looking at the book. This is just to see how well you have understood and can recall the information presented in this chapter after you have studied it and completed the workbook exercises. You will not be graded on this portion (other than the grade you give yourself), but this is an excellent preparation for your instructor's test. You may use this Post-Test to determine what areas you need to study more. Justify any "false" answers.

1. Medical insurance coding is a way of putting procedures and treatments into numeric form. (T or F)

2. CPT stands for:
   a. Comprehensive Procedural Terminology
   b. Current Procedural Terminology
   c. Complete Procedural Terminology
   d. Curative Procedural Terminology

3. ICD stands for:
   a. International Codes for Diagnosis
   b. Internal Codes for Diagnosis
   c. International Codes for Diseases
   d. International Classifications of Diseases

4. Third-party guidelines have the expectation that insurance companies will not disclose personal medical information to unauthorized persons. (T or F)

5. Insurance coding, claim forms, and submissions are complex enough that medical coders and billers need extended training and experience to do it well. (T or F)

CERTIFICATION CRITERIA CHECKLIST

As you go through your education and training, keep in mind the national certification examination that you will take when you graduate. Each chapter of the textbook and workbook covers a different section of the examination criteria. To keep track of your preparation for the certification examination, turn to the back of this workbook and highlight the following CMA, RMA, or CMAS certification examination criteria (if you have already highlighted them from a previous chapter, put a check mark by the criteria):

CMA
F. Medicolegal Guidelines & Requirements
    5. Physician–patient relationship
Q. Managing Practice Finances
    2. Coding systems

RMA

II.   Administrative Medical Assisting

    A.   Insurance

CMAS

5.   Health Care Insurance Processing, Coding and Billing

    •   Insurance coding

COMPETENCY ASSESSMENT
Procedure 19-1 Current Procedural Terminology Coding

Performance Objectives: To convert commonly accepted descriptions of medical procedures (services) and for visits of all kinds—office, hospital, nursing facility, home services—into a five-digit numeric code with two-digit numeric modifiers when required. Perform this objective within 15 minutes with a minimum score of 15 points.

Supplies/Equipment: CPT code book for the current year, copy of the encounter form and access to the patient's chart, pencil and paper

Charting/Documentation: Enter appropriate documentation/charting in the box.

Instructor's/Evaluator's Comments and Suggestions:

SKILLS CHECKLIST Procedure 19-1: Current Procedural Terminology Coding

Name _____

Date _____

No.	Skill	Check #1 20 pts ea	Check #2 10 pts ea	Check #3 5 pts ea	Notes
1	Using the CPT code book, look in the Evaluation and Management section, Office or Other Outpatient Services, New Patient. Read through until the code matching the described scenario is found.				
2	Look up Urinalysis, Routine in CPT code book index.				
3	Locate code 81002 in the Pathology and Laboratory section. Be sure the description provided matches what the physician has documented in the patient chart.				
Student's Total Points					
Points Possible		60	30	15	
Final Score (Student's Total Points / Possible Points)					

Notes

Start time:

End time:

Total time: (15 min goal)

COMPETENCY ASSESSMENT

Procedure 19-2 International Classification of Diseases, 9th Revision, Clinical Modification Coding

Performance Objectives: The ICD-9-CM code books provide a diagnostic coding system for the compilation and reporting of morbidity and mortality statistics for reimbursement purposes. Perform this objective within 15 minutes with a minimum score of 10 points.

Supplies/Equipment: Volumes 1 and 2 of the ICD-9-CM code books for the current year, copy of the encounter form and access to the patient's chart, pencil and paper

Charting/Documentation: Enter appropriate documentation/charting in the box.

_____

_____

_____

_____

Instructor's/Evaluator's Comments and Suggestions:

_____

_____

_____

_____

_____

SKILLS CHECKLIST Procedure 19-2: International Classification of Diseases, 9th Revision, Clinical Modification Coding

Name _____

Date _____

No.	Skill	Check #1 20 pts ea	Check #2 10 pts ea	Check #3 5 pts ea	Notes
1	Using Volume II of the ICD-9-CM code books, look up the main reason or condition that brought the patient to the facility, or the specific diagnosis confirmed by test results (code 599.0).				
2	Using Volume I, look up code 599. Read all 599 listings and determine the appropriate code having the greatest level of specificity.				
Student's Total Points					
Points Possible		40	20	10	
Final Score (Student's Total Points / Possible Points)					

	Notes
Start time:	
End time:	
Total time: (15 min goal)	

COMPETENCY ASSESSMENT

Procedure 19-3 Applying Third-Party Guidelines

Performance Objectives: To obtain written authorization to release necessary medical information to third-party payers. Perform this objective within 5 minutes with a minimum score of 10 points.

Supplies/Equipment: Patient chart, CMS-1500 claim form

Charting/Documentation: Enter appropriate documentation/charting in the box.

_____

_____

_____

_____

Instructor's/Evaluator's Comments and Suggestions:

_____

_____

_____

_____

_____

_____

SKILLS CHECKLIST Procedure 19-3: Applying Third-Party Guidelines

Name _____

Date _____

No.	Skill	Check #1 20 pts ea	Check #2 10 pts ea	Check #3 5 pts ea	Notes
1	When patient signs in, check their chart to ascertain if an "Authorization to Release Medical Information" has been signed and is currently valid.				
2	If there is no record of signature on file, have the patient sign Block 12 of the CMS-1500 form.				
	Student's Total Points				
	Points Possible	40	20	10	
	Final Score (Student's Total Points / Possible Points)				

	Notes
Start time:	
End time:	
Total time: (5 min goal)	

COMPETENCY ASSESSMENT

Procedure 19-4 Completing a Medicare CMS-1500 Claim Form

Performance Objectives: To complete the CMS-1500 insurance claim form for Medicare for Reimbursement. Perform this objective within 30 minutes with a minimum score of 270 points.

Supplies/Equipment: Patient information, patient account or ledger card, copy of patient's insurance card, insurance claim form, computer and printer.

Charting/Documentation: Enter appropriate documentation/charting in the box.

_____

_____

_____

_____

Instructor's/Evaluator's Comments and Suggestions:

_____

_____

_____

_____

_____

_____

SKILLS CHECKLIST Procedure 19-4: Completing a Medicare CMS-1500 Claim Form

Name _____

Date _____

No.	Skill	Check #1 20 pts ea	Check #2 10 pts ea	Check #3 5 pts ea	Notes
1	Key in the carrier's name and address if it is not already imprinted.				
2	Complete each block as directed in the patient and insured information section.				
	Block 1 — Applicable health insurance coverage				
	Block 2 — Patient name				
	Block 3 — Birth date and sex				
	Block 5 — Mailing address and telephone number				
	Block 6 — Relationship to insured				
	Block 8 — Marital status and employment or school status				
	Blocks 9a, 9b, 9c — Completed if patient has Medigap				
	Block 10 — Indicate if condition related to work or accident				
	Block 10d — Medicaid information if appropriate				
	Block 12 — Signature of patient or representative				
3	Complete the Insured Information section:				
	Block 1a — HICN				
	Block 4 — Other insurance primary?				
	Block 7 — Insured's address and telephone number				
	Block 11— If other insurance is primary, enter group number				
	Block 11a — Insured's birth date and sex				
	Block 11b — Insured's employer's name				
	Block 11c — Primary insured's payer identification (ID) number or plan name				
	Block 11d — Blank				
	Block 13 — Signature of insured				

No.	Skill	Check #1 20 pts ea	Check #2 10 pts ea	Check #3 5 pts ea	Notes
4	Physician or supplier information:				
	Block 14 — Patient's date of illness or injury				
	Block 15 — Blank				
	Block 17 — Name of referring physician or ordering physician (if supplied)				
	Block 17a — UPIN of referring or ordering physician				
	Block 19 — Date patient last seen and UPIN of attending physician				
	Block 21 — Patient's diagnosis code				
	Block 24A — Date for each procedure, service, or supply				
	Block 24B — Place of service code				
	Block 24C — Blank for Medicare providers				
	Block 24D — CPT codes				
	Block 24E — Diagnostic codes related to the DOS and the procedures				
	Block 25 — Provider's Federal Tax ID number				
	Block 26 — Patient's account number				
	Block 27 — Accept assignment?				
	Block 31 — Signature of provider				
	Block 32 — Name and address of provider facility				
5	Complete the physician or supplier information:				
	Block 16 — Date patient is unable to work				
	Block 18 — Date medical service is furnished if related to hospitalization				
	Block 20 — Complete when billing for tests subject to price limits				
	Block 22 — Blank				
	Block 23 — Prior authorization number if required				
	Block 24F — Charge for each service				

No.	Skill	Check #1 20 pts ea	Check #2 10 pts ea	Check #3 5 pts ea	Notes
	Block 24G — Number of days or units if applicable				
	Block 24H — Blank				
	Block 24I — Blank				
	Block 24J — Blank				
	Block 24K — Pin number of provider				
	Block 28 — Total charges				
	Block 29 — Total paid by patient				
	Block 30 — Blank				
	Block 33 — Providers billing name, address, and phone number				
Student's Total Points					
Points Possible (54 steps)		1080	540	270	
Final Score (Student's Total Points / Possible Points)					
		Notes			
Start time:					
End time:					
Total time: (30 min goal)					

EVALUATION OF CHAPTER KNOWLEDGE

Skills	Student Self-Evaluation		
	Good	Average	Poor
I understand the process of procedure and diagnosis coding.	____	____	____
I can code a sample claim form.	____	____	____
I document accurately.	____	____	____
I can explain the difference between the CMS-1500 and the UB92 forms.	____	____	____
I can describe ways in which computers have altered the claims processes.	____	____	____
I can discuss why claims follow-up is important to the ambulatory care setting.	____	____	____
I can discuss the legal and ethical issues associated with insurance coding.	____	____	____
I am comfortable as a patient educator about insurance issues.	____	____	____

CHAPTER 20

Billing and Collections

CHAPTER PRE-TEST

Perform this test without looking at the book. This is just to see how well you have understood and can recall the information in this chapter after you have read it, but before you have completed the workbook exercises. You will not be graded on this portion (other than the grade you give yourself). Justify any "false" answers.

1. The Truth-in-Lending Act states:
   a. Physicians cannot charge more than 10% interest on their patient accounts.
   b. Physicians must charge interest if the account is more than 4 months past due.
   c. Physicians must notify the patients in writing if interest is to be charged on their accounts.
   d. If the physician and patient agree to an installation plan of more than four payments, the installation charge must be stated in writing.

2. The best opportunity for collection is at the time of services. (T or F)

3. Large clinics with numerous statements to send out each month will find the monthly billing cycle method to be the most efficient. (T or F)

4. A collection ratio of 80% is considered a good ratio. (T or F)

INTRODUCTION

Accurate and timely patient billing is essential to maintaining the financial health of an ambulatory care facility. Medical assistants play a vital role in managing accounts receivable. Establishing and monitoring patient billing, using either a manual or computerized system, requires attention to detail, accurate documentation, and excellent communication skills when performing duties related to the collection of outstanding debt. When performing billing and collection tasks, it is important to remember that patients have the right to choose their health care providers and should be respected as consumers.

PERFORMANCE OBJECTIVES

After successful completion of this chapter you will be able to explain the terminology related to medical billing and collections. You will be able to analyze the importance of billing accurately and billing (at least collecting copayment) at the time of services, differentiate between monthly and cycle billing, recall the components of a complete statement, analyze the importance of correct telephone collection process, and explain the process of aging accounts. You will be able to discuss the Truth-in-Lending Act, compare manual billing with computerized billing, and recall points to consider when using a collection agency. You will also be able to recall special collections problems encountered in the ambulatory care setting, describe the process of sending a collection letter, explain the ramifications of the statute of limitations, and explain the merits of a professional attitude when handling collections. *The following statements are related to your learning objectives for this chapter. Fill in the blanks in the following paragraph with the appropriate term(s).*

The ambulatory care setting's cash flow and collection process are dependent on (1) _____. The (2) _____ status of the practice is reflected in the unpaid balance of the patient accounts. The best opportunity for collection, especially of the copayment amounts, is (3) _____. The (4) _____ states that a practice must clearly define the charges and the interest being charged when installation payments (four or more) are being arranged with a patient. Collection letters are usually sent after (5) _____ statements have been sent to the patient with no response. When using a collection agency, the following questions should be asked: (6) _____, (7) _____, (8) _____, (9) _____, (10) _____, and (11) _____. The difference between accounts receivable ratio and collection ratio is that the (12) _____ refers to the speed at which the outstanding accounts are paid, and the (13) _____ _____ shows the status of the paid accounts and possible losses. Three special collection situations encountered in the ambulatory care setting are (14) _____, (15) _____, and (16) _____. The (17) _____ defines the period in which legal action may take place.

VOCABULARY BUILDER

Find the words below that are misspelled; circle them, and then correctly spell them in the spaces provided. Then match each correct vocabulary term to its definition below.

accounts recievable ratio   collection agency   Statute of limatations

aging accounts   collection ratio   Truth-in-Lending Act

cicyle billing   monthly billing

_____   _____   _____

1. _____ A method that sends all bills at the same time each month, usually on or about the 25th day of each month

2. _____ A process by which accounts are determined to be overdue

3. _____ Also known as the Consumer Credit Protection Act of 1968; an act requiring providers of installment credits to state the charges in writing and to express the interest as an annual rate

4. _____ An outside establishment that collects outstanding debt

5. _____ Statute that defines the period of time in which legal action can take place

6. _____ A method of spreading billing over the whole month instead of sending bills at the end of the month

7. _____ The status of collections and the possible losses in a medical facility

8. _____ Measures the speed with which outstanding accounts are paid

LEARNING REVIEW

1. A billing efficiency report allows for careful monitoring of follow-up bills; that is, whether they were paid, if the insurance has paid, and an assessment of the patient's responsibility for payment. What five pieces of data are included in these reports from which production efficiency is calculated?

   (1) _____   (4) _____

   (2) _____   (5) _____

   (3) _____

2. Identify and explain the five most common reasons some patient accounts become past due.

   (1) _____

   (2) _____

   (3) _____

   (4) _____

   (5) _____

3. A. In the pegboard system, what method is used to identify the age of accounts?

   _____

   _____

   B. A written code "OD2/ 4/1" is entered on a patient ledger card. What does the code mean?

   _____

   C. Name five criteria according to which computer programs can age accounts.

   (1) _____   (4) _____

   (2) _____   (5) _____

   (3) _____

   D. The computer can also generate accounts receivable reports. Name three pieces of information included on a computer-generated accounts receivable report.

   (1) _____

   (2) _____

   (3) _____

4. Collection agencies generally provide two services to an ambulatory care facility. Name and describe each type of service.

   (1) _____

   _____

   (2) _____

   _____

5. Collection of fees when a patient has died are directed to the executor of the estate. Place a check mark next to each action below that represents a responsible action in collecting past due accounts from deceased patients' estates.

   ____ A. If there is no known administrator, address the statement to "Estate of (insert patient's name)" and mail to the patient's last known address.

   ____ B. Send an invoice via certified mail with a complete breakdown of all monies owed by the deceased patient's spouse or closest relative, noting that the survivor is responsible for making payment in full.

   ____ C. Wait a minimum of 10 days after the death to send a statement to the estate, out of respect for the family of the deceased.

   ____ D. If unsure how to proceed, contact the office's attorney or the probate court for advice on how to proceed.

6. With regard to collections, the statute of limitations is usually defined by the class of the overdue account. Name the three classes of accounts.

   (1) _____

   (2) _____

   (3) _____

7. The most appropriate time to discuss fees with patients is when:
   a. services are rendered
   b. scheduling the first appointment
   c. sent by mail after services are rendered
   d. the insurance company does not pay the fee

8. The Truth-in-Lending Act is also known as the:
   a. Consumer Credit Protection Act
   b. Fair Debt Collection Practice Act
   c. Patient Bankruptcy Protection Act
   d. Accurate Billing and Collection Act

9. The charge slip is also known as the:
   a. ledger
   b. encounter form
   c. day sheet
   d. CMS-1500

10. When a patient files for bankruptcy:
    a. there is little likelihood that the debt can be collected
    b. it is best to close the account and identify the loss
    c. file a proof of claim and a copy of the account to the bankruptcy court
    d. take the account to small claims court

11. In determining how aggressive to be in debt collections, you should consider:
    a. the previous month's billing backlog
    b. production efficiency
    c. the terms of the insured's policy
    d. the value of the dollar owed

CERTIFICATION REVIEW

These questions are designed to mimic the certification examinations. You can use these questions like a small "Certification Examination Study Guide," but this is not meant to take the place of the more extensive study guides. Use this portion to determine in what areas to concentrate your efforts when studying for the certification examination. Justify any "false" answers.

1. Most states limit collections calls to between 8 AM and 8 PM. (T or F)

2. Emancipated minors are responsible for their own accounts. (T or F)

3. Collection agencies must abide by different rules than the ambulatory care center. (T or F)

4. Patients who owe money but have moved and left no forwarding address are referred to as:

   a. deadbeats

   b. skips

   c. nonpayers

   d. dead accounts

5. Statutes of limitations vary from state to state, but are usually:

   a. up to 3 years

   b. 5–10 years

   c. up to 10 years

   d. without a time limit if the account is more than a certain amount

CASE STUDY

Charles Williams, 62 years old, is a new patient of Dr. Winston Lewis at the offices of Drs. Lewis and King. On July 1, 20XX, 5 days before the patient's birthday, Charles comes to see Dr. Lewis for an appointment with a chief complaint of intermittent, irregular heartbeats or palpitations, dizziness, and chest pain. Dr. Lewis performs a comprehensive physical examination and orders several tests, including an EKG, complete blood count (CBC), and urinalysis with microscopy. The total fee for the office visit and tests is $345: $200 for the physical examination, $75 for the EKG, $25 for the urinalysis, $25 for routine venipuncture, and $20 for a CBC, which Charles pays for by check at the time of service. Charles is insured by a private carrier, All American Insurance Company, group #333210, ID number 112-45-9980, which he receives through his employer, HighTech Computer Group. Dr. Lewis asks Ellen Armstrong, CMA, to schedule a return appointment in exactly one week to go over the results of Charles's tests. Ellen schedules the appointment and prepares a charge slip for Charles's visit. She refers to his patient information sheet for the correct personal information. Charles Williams lives at 123 Greenside Street, Northborough, OH, 12346.

Complete the charge slip for Charles Williams' office visit (Figure 20-1).

SELF-ASSESSMENT

Think about a time or times when you had paid a bill late or not paid it until the following month. Without disclosing too much personal information, answer the following:

1. What was your reason(s)?

2. Did you receive an overdue notice or a phone call?

3. Which do you think would be more difficult to receive?

4. Are you likely to become defensive if the caller or notice has a threatening tone or a more understanding tone?

5. Could the tone of the notice/call leave you feeling good/bad about the event?

6. Think of ways the situation could have been handled better.

7. Will your experience affect the way you treat people who owe your clinic money?

DATE	PATIENT	SERVICE CODE	FEES CHARGE	PAID	ADJ.	BALANCE DUE	PREVIOUS BALANCE	NAME	RECEIPT NO.
				CREDITS					

THIS IS YOUR RECEIPT _____
AND/OR A STATEMENT OF YOUR ACCOUNT TO DATE _____

PATIENT'S NAME ☐ M ☐ F

ADDRESS

CITY   STATE   ZIP

OFFICE VISITS AND PROCEDURES

99211	EST PT - MINIMAL OV	1				HOSPITAL VISIT	14
99212	EST PT - BRIEF OV	2				EMERGENCY	15
99213	EST PT - INTERMEDIATE OV	3				CONSULTATION	16
99214	EST PT - EXTENDED OV	4		93000		EKG	17
99215	EST PT - COMPREHENSIVE OV	5		93224		ELECTROCARDIOGRAPHIC MONITORING	18
99201	NEW PT - BRIEF OV	6		93307		ECHOCARDIOGRAPHY	19
99202	NEW PT - INTERMEDIATE OV	7		85025		CBC	20
99203	NEW PT - EXTENDED OV	8		81000		URINALYSIS WITH MICROSCOPY	21
99204	NEW PT - COMPLEX OV	9		36415		ROUTINE VENIPUNCTURE	22
99205	NEW PT - COMPREHENSIVE OF	10		71020		RADIOLOGY EXAM-CHEST-2 VIEWS	23
99238	HOSPITAL DISCHARGE	11		30300		REMOVE FOR. BODY-INTRANASAL	24
99025	NEW PT - SURGERY PROC. PRIMARY	12					25
	NURSING HOME VISIT	13					26

RELATIONSHIP   BIRTHDATE

SUBSCRIBER OR POLICY HOLDER

☐ MEDICARE ☐ MEDICAID ☐ BLUE SHIELD ☐ 65-SP.

INSURANCE CARRIER

AGREEMENT #

GROUP #

D - OTHER SERVICES

AUTHORIZATION TO RELEASE INFORMATION: I HEREBY AUTHORIZE THE UNDERSIGNED PHYSICIAN TO RELEASE ANY INFORMATION ACQUIRED IN THE COURSE OF MY EXAMINATION OR TREATMENT.
SIGNED (PATIENT, OR PARENT IF MINOR)

_____ DATE _____

NEXT APPOINTMENT _____ AT _____ AM PM
RETURN _____ DAYS _____ WEEKS _____ MONTHS

PLACE OF SERVICE ☐ OFFICE ☐ OTHER _____

DIAGNOSIS OR SYMPTOMS _____

DOCTOR'S SIGNATURE _____

L&K LEWIS & KING, MD
2501 CENTER STREET
NORTHBOROUGH, OH 12345

03626

Figure 20-1

CHAPTER POST-TEST

This is similar to the Pre-Test. Perform this test without looking at the book. This is just to see how well you have understood and can recall the information presented in this chapter after you have studied it and completed the workbook exercises. You will not be graded on this portion (other than the grade you give yourself), but this is an excellent preparation for your instructor's test. You may use this Post-Test to determine what areas you need to study more. Justify any "false" answers.

1. The Truth-in-Lending Act states:
   a. Physicians can charge more than 10% interest on their patient accounts.
   b. Physicians can only charge interest if the account is more than 4 months overdue.
   c. Physicians must notify patients in person if interest is to be charged on their accounts.
   d. If the physician and patient agree to an installation plan of more than four payments, the installation charge must be stated in writing.

2. The best opportunity for collection is within 30 days of the time of service. (T or F)

3. Large clinics with numerous statements to send out each month will find the cycle billing method to be the most efficient. (T or F)

4. A collection ratio of 90% is considered a good ratio. (T or F)

CERTIFICATION CRITERIA CHECKLIST

As you go through your education and training, keep in mind the national certification examination that you will take when you graduate. Each chapter of the textbook and workbook covers a different section of the examination criteria. To keep track of your preparation for the certification examination turn to the back of this workbook and highlight the following CMA, RMA, or CMAS certification examination criteria (if you have already highlighted them from a previous chapter, put a check mark by the criteria):

CMA
E. Communication
    4. Professional communication and behavior
F. Medicolegal Guidelines & Requirements
    2. Legislation
Q. Managing Practice Finances
    1. Bookkeeping systems
    4. Accounting and banking procedures

RMA
II. Administrative Medical Assisting
    B. Finance/Bookkeeping

CMAS
6. Medical Office Financial Management
    • Fundamentals of financial management
    • Patient accounts

COMPETENCY ASSESSMENT

Procedure 20-1 Explaining Fees in the First Telephone Interview

Performance Objectives: To establish rapport with patients; to discuss physicians' fees; to identify patient responsibility before the first visit. Perform this objective within 15 minutes with a minimum score of 50 points.

Supplies/Equipment: Physician's fee schedule, appointment schedule, telephone

Charting/Documentation: Enter appropriate documentation/charting in the box.

_____

_____

_____

_____

Instructor's/Evaluator's Comments and Suggestions:

_____

_____

_____

_____

_____

_____

SKILLS CHECKLIST Procedure 20-1: Explaining Fees in the First Telephone Interview

Name _____

Date _____

No.	Skill	Check #1 20 pts ea	Check #2 10 pts ea	Check #3 5 pts ea	Notes
1	Place the physician's fee schedule and the appointment schedule close to the telephone.				
2	Answer call before the third ring. Identify name of the clinic and yourself.				
3	Offer assistance.				
4	Determine nature of visit, and if patient is new. Discuss possible dates for the appointment.				
5	Tell the patient you will be discussing clinic policies and will mail the Patient Information Brochure before the appointment.				
6	Ask about medical insurance. Get the identification number, name of subscriber, employer, and a telephone number of carrier.				
7	Explain that any copayment and coinsurance will be due at the time of visit.				
8	Check to see if the patient has transportation and knows how to get to the clinic. Provide directions if needed.				
9	Request that the patient arrive 15 minutes early to complete forms.				
10	After closing interview, promptly mail the Patient Information Brochure.				
Student's Total Points					
Points Possible		200	100	50	
Final Score (Student's Total Points / Possible Points)					

	Notes
Start time:	
End time:	
Total time: (15 min goal)	

COMPETENCY ASSESSMENT

Procedure 20-2 Prepare Itemized Patient Accounts for Billing

Performance Objectives: To notify patients of the fees for services rendered and collect on those accounts. Perform this objective within 20 minutes with a minimum score of 50 points.

Supplies/Equipment: Computer or typewriter, calculator, patient account of ledger cards, billing statement forms

Charting/Documentation: Enter appropriate documentation/charting in the box.

_____

_____

_____

_____

Instructor's/Evaluator's Comments and Suggestions:

_____

_____

_____

_____

_____

SKILLS CHECKLIST Procedure 20-2: Prepare Itemized Patient Accounts for Billing

Name _____

Date _____

No.	Skill	Check #1 20 pts ea	Check #2 10 pts ea	Check #3 5 pts ea	Notes
1	Gather all accounts and ledgers with outstanding balances.				
2	Separate any accounts that are labeled as past due.				
	a. For each account, verify name and address of patient and person responsible for payment.				
	b. Place current date on statement.				
	c. Scan account information for errors.				
	d. Itemize procedures in layman's terms and indicate charges.				
	e. Identify and subtract any payments.				
	f. Calculate the unpaid balance.				
3	Discuss with the office manager and follow through on any action to be taken on past-due accounts.				
4	Place statements in envelopes and mail.				
Student's Total Points					
Points Possible (10 steps total)		200	100	50	
Final Score (Student's Total Points / Possible Points)					

	Notes
Start time:	
End time:	
Total time: (20 min goal)	

COMPETENCY ASSESSMENT

Procedure 20-3 Post/Record Adjustments

Performance Objectives: To keep track of financial adjustments. Perform this objective within 15 minutes with a minimum score of 20 points.

Supplies/Equipment: Computerized or manual bookkeeping system, patient's account, black or blue and red pen for use in manual bookkeeping system

Charting/Documentation: Enter appropriate documentation/charting in the box.

_____

_____

_____

_____

Instructor's/Evaluator's Comments and Suggestions:

_____

_____

_____

_____

_____

_____

SKILLS CHECKLIST Procedure 20-3: Post/Record Adjustments

Name _____

Date _____

No.	Skill	Check #1 20 pts ea	Check #2 10 pts ea	Check #3 5 pts ea	Notes
1	With the daily schedule of services/charges before you, enter amount received from the collection agency on a patient's account with an explanation note.				
2	Record the amount received and the explanation in the patient's account.				
3	Subtract the amount paid by the collection agency from the total charges to create the new balance.				
4	Write off this balance, indicating a zero balance on the patient's account. The difference between the amount collected and amount paid by the agency is entered as a negative adjustment on the daily sheet.				
Student's Total Points					
Points Possible		80	40	20	
Final Score (Student's Total Points / Possible Points)					

	Notes
Start time:	
End time:	
Total time: (15 min goal)	

EVALUATION OF CHAPTER KNOWLEDGE

Skills	Student Self-Evaluation		
	Good	Average	Poor
I understand credit and collection policies and procedures.	_____	_____	_____
I understand the process of aging accounts.	_____	_____	_____
I recognize components of a complete patient statement.	_____	_____	_____
I can accurately complete a charge slip.	_____	_____	_____
I possess the ability to hold a professional telephone collection call.	_____	_____	_____
I can identify collection techniques and describe the use of each.	_____	_____	_____
I possess the ability to compose collection letters.	_____	_____	_____
I understand the importance of accounts receivable to the financial health of the ambulatory care setting.	_____	_____	_____
I know the function of credit bureaus and collection agencies.	_____	_____	_____
I can identify special collection situations and strategies for handling them.	_____	_____	_____
I can consider legal ramifications of billing and collection procedures, including the Truth-in-Lending Act, Fair Debt Collection Practices Act, small claims court, and the statute of limitations.	_____	_____	_____

CHAPTER 21

Accounting Practices

CHAPTER PRE-TEST

Perform this test without looking at the book. This is just to see how well you have understood and can recall the information in this chapter after you have read it, but before you have completed the workbook exercises. You will not be graded on this portion (other than the grade you give yourself). Justify any "false" answers.

1. Accounts receivable is the amount the physician is owed by patients. (T or F)

2. The purpose of cost analysis is to:
   a. determine the costs of each service
   b. determine the fixed costs
   c. determine the variable costs
   d. determine the total of all of the above

3. Income statements should show both profits and expenses. (T or F)

4. The W-4 Form shows the employee's withholding allowance. (T or F)

INTRODUCTION

The management of practice finances in the ambulatory care setting is one of the most important aspects in the operation of the facility. The proper management of medical facility finances includes daily financial practices, the accurate coding and processing of insurance forms, collection of accounts, and accounting practices. Accounting in the ambulatory care setting includes the collection of data on all aspects of the financial operation. If done properly, accounting can monitor the profitability of a facility and ensure that any new activities, such as computerization, result in optimum financial health. The administrative duties of medical assistants will require them to become involved in the financial operations of the ambulatory care setting. A working knowledge of accounting processes will also help medical assistants become aware of the manner in which financial realities influence workplace decisions in the ambulatory care setting, such as purchasing new equipment, hiring new employees, or implementing a facility newsletter for community outreach and patient education.

PERFORMANCE OBJECTIVES

After successful completion of this chapter you will be able to explain the terminology related to medical accounting practices used in ambulatory settings. You will be able to describe four different types of bookkeeping and accounting systems, and compare and contrast financial, managerial, and cost accounting. You will be able to explain the use and validity of the income statement, the balance sheet, the day-end summary, and the accounts receivable trial balance, as well as recall and explain useful financial ratios. You will be able to identify proper steps in accounts payable management and the impact of utilization review on reimbursement. You will also become well aware of the legal and ethical guidelines in accounting practices. *The following statements are related to your learning objectives for this chapter. Fill in the blanks in the following paragraph with the appropriate term(s).*

Accounting generates (1) _____ information for the office. Although

there are several different types of bookkeeping systems available to the office, most are going

away from manual accounting systems and more toward (2) _____

systems. (3) _____ accounting provides information primarily for

entities external to the clinic, such as for government. (4) _____

accounting generates financial information that can enable more efficient internal control.

(5) _____ accounting helps to determine what price the ambulatory care

office is paying to perform particular services. The financial summary at the end of the day is called

the (6) _____. The (7) _____

_____ will indicate any problem

between the daily journal and the ledger. Cost analysis is used to determine the costs of

(8) _____. (9) _____ costs are those expenses that do

not vary in total as the number of the patients vary. By contrast, the (10) _____

_____ costs vary according to patient volume. The most commonly generated year-end

report is called a (11) _____. A balance sheet is sometimes called a

(12) _____ and

is an itemized statement of (13) _____, (14) _____, and

the (15) _____ as of a

specific date. Ratios are not difficult to calculate but can be (16) _____

_____ when using a manual system. The accounts receivable ratio measures

the (17) _____, the collection

ratio shows the (18) _____, and the

cost ratio shows the (19) _____.

VOCABULARY BUILDER

Find the words below that are misspelled; circle them, and then correctly spell them in the spaces provided. Then match each definition below to its correct vocabulary term.

_____ 1. accounting

_____ 2. accounts payible

_____ 3. accounts recievable ratio

_____ 4. assets

_____ 5. balance sheet

_____ 6. collection ratio

_____ 7. check register

_____ 8. cost analalysis

_____ 9. cost ratio

_____ 10. cash bases of accounting

_____ 11. fixed costs

_____ 12. income statement

_____ 13. libilities

_____ 14. accrual basis of accounting

_____ 15. owner's equity

_____ 16. utilazation review

_____ 17. varieble costs

_____

_____

_____

_____

_____

_____

A. Financial statement showing net profit or loss

B. These vary in direct proportion to patient volume

C. Records and categorizes all checks written

D. The outstanding accounts receivable divided by the average monthly gross income for the past 12 months

E. A procedure that determines the cost of each service

F. An itemized statement of assets, liabilities, financial condition, and owner's equity

G. Income is recognized when the money is collected

H. These do not vary in total as the number of patients varies

I. System of monitoring the financial status of a facility and the financial results of its activities, providing information for decision making

J. Debts, financial obligations, for which one is responsible

K. The gross income divided by the amount that could have been collected, less adjustments

L. Properties of value that are owned by a business entity

M. An unwritten promise to pay a supplier for property or merchandise purchased on credit or for a service rendered

N. The amount by which business assets exceed business liabilities

O. Formula that shows the cost of a procedure or service and helps determine the financial value of maintaining certain services

P. Reports income at the time charges are generated

Q. A review of medical services before they can be performed

LEARNING REVIEW

1. There are a variety of methods used for financial management in the ambulatory care setting. Name three bookkeeping systems that are appropriate for use in a noncomputerized, or manual, environment.

   (1) _____

   (2) _____

   (3) _____

   Match the appropriate bookkeeping system to the following duties performed by the medical assistant.

   _____ A. Office manager Walter Seals, CMA, was responsible for implementing a computer system at Inner City Health Care. Before the computerized accounting program was put into effect, the urgent care center relied on a manual system of checks and balances that allowed the physician–employers to keep a firm hold on the relation between the facility's assets and the sum of liabilities and net worth.

   _____ B. During a temporary one-week down period in the computer system at the offices of Drs. Lewis and King while a system upgrade is installed, administrative medical assistant Ellen Armstrong completes each day's financial transactions in a daily journal, then transfers this information to the ledger through the posting process. The information will be entered into the computer once the system is up and running again.

   _____ C. When the patient returns the charge slip to the reception desk after an examination, Karen Ritter, CMA, carefully replaces and lines up the charge slip with the patient's name on the day sheet, then correctly inserts the ledger card under the last page of the charge slip. She proceeds to enter the total charges due and any patient payments.

2. A. Medical software packages have the ability to code information obtained in the ambulatory care setting for use in a database. When completing insurance claim forms or generating reports, the software has the capability to include the most common _____ and _____ codes. What other kinds of codes can a computerized accounting system generate that will facilitate the billing functions?

   _____

   _____

   _____

   B. The computer can also be used in the preparation of financial documents. Name four financial documents.

   (1) _____

   (2) _____

   (3) _____

   (4) _____

3. Name three ways computer service bureaus handle accounts from medical facilities.

   (1) _____

   _____

   (2) _____

   _____

   (3) _____

   _____

4. Identify at least four steps to take to reduce the chance of embezzlement.

   (1) _____

   (2) _____

   (3) _____

   (4) _____

5. Fixed costs are expenses that do not vary in total as the number of patients seen by the medical practice grows or shrinks. Variable costs are expenses that are directly affected by patient volume.

   From the list below, identify expenses that qualify as fixed costs (FC) and those that are variable costs (VC).

   _____ 1. Interpreting laboratory test results

   _____ 2. Annual depreciation of the cost of an automatic electrocardiograph (ECG) machine

   _____ 3. Medical benefits for the office staff

   _____ 4. Purchase of reagent test strips for urinalysis

   _____ 5. Magazine subscriptions for the facility reception area

   _____ 6. Monthly telephone expenses

   _____ 7. Medical journal subscriptions for the physician–owners

   _____ 8. Purchase of a HemoCue blood glucose system

   _____ 9. Printing cost of a patient education brochure

   _____ 10. Purchase of open-shelf lateral files

   _____ 11. Adding a new position, such as a clinical medical assistant, to the office staff

   _____ 12. Property taxes on the medical facility building and grounds

   _____ 13. The monthly cost of janitorial services

   _____ 14. Purchase of disposable needle-syringe units

   _____ 15. Disposable paper gowns for patient examinations

6. To protect the practice from financial loss, physicians can purchase fidelity bonds. Name and describe the three kinds of bonds. Place a check mark in front of the one that offers the most assurance.

   (1) _____

   (2) _____

   (3) _____

7. At the offices of Drs. Lewis and King, the total accounts receivable at the end of May is $100,000 and the monthly receipts total is $75,000; the total accounts receivable at the end of June is $82,000 and the monthly receipts total is $31,000; the total accounts receivable at the end of July is $86,000 and the monthly receipts total is $20,000; the total accounts receivable at the end of August is $93,000 and the monthly receipts total is $15,000. What is the accounts receivable ratio for each month? Show your calculations in the space provided.

   May: July:

   June: August:

   Which month has the healthiest accounts receivable ratio? Why?

   _____

8. A. For the month of September, receipts at the offices of Drs. Lewis and King totaled $35,000. The Medicare/Medicaid adjustment for the month was $1,750, and the managed care adjustment was $4,500. Total charges for the month of September equaled $53,000. What is the collection ratio for the month of September? Show your calculation in the space provided.

   _____

   _____

   B. For the month of October, receipts at the offices of Drs. Lewis and King totaled $41,000. The Medicare/Medicaid adjustment for the month was $2,000, the Worker's Compensation adjustment was $750, and the managed care adjustment was $4,700. Total charges for October equaled $55,000. What is the collection ratio for the month of October? Show your calculation in the space provided.

   _____

   _____

   C. Which month has the more desirable collection ratio? Why?

   _____

9. A. A group practice of radiologists charges $225 for a routine mammogram. Total expenses related to the mammogram procedure equal $30,000 per month, and the practice performs a monthly average of 200 mammograms. What is the average cost ratio for the mammogram procedure? Show your calculations in the space provided.

   _____

   _____

B. Given the cost to patients for the mammogram procedure, is the group practice making a profit or loss on performing mammograms? What amount is the profit or loss per procedure? What amount is the profit or loss for the entire month?

_____

_____

10. A. Income statements reveal the cumulative profit and total expenses for each month. Monthly income and expenses are then added to arrive at year-to-date totals, which are compared with the annual budget for particular income and expense categories. Use the following information to complete the expense analysis for the first quarter office expense costs of the offices of Drs. Lewis and King. The total office expense budget for the year is $20,000 divided evenly per quarter.

Telephone expenses for January = $323.46, February = $425.93, March = $393.87

Postage and mail expenses for January = $725.45, February = $550.90, March = $601.33

Office supply expenses for January = $1,200.62, February = $325.45, March = $446.26

Yearly budget for telephone expenses = $4,000, postage and mail expenses = $8,000, office supply expenses = $8,000

Office Expenses	January	February	March	Year-to-Date	Budget for Year
Office supplies	$	$	$	$	$
Postage	$	$	$	$	$
Telephone	$	$	$	$	$
TOTALS	**$**	**$**	**$**	**$**	**$**

B. How much are the offices of Drs. Lewis and King over or under budget for quarterly office expenses? _____ How might the office manager use data from the budget sheet?

_____

_____

Why is it important to implement and track budgets for specific categories of income and expense in the ambulatory care setting?

_____

_____

11. Financial records should provide the following at all times:
    a. salaries earned by physicians and staff
    b. amount earned, owed, and collected within a given period
    c. where expenses incurred in a given period
    d. b and c

12. A hospital cost report for Medicare is a part of:
    a. financial accounting
    b. managerial accounting
    c. cost accounting
    d. cost analysis

13. Examples of variable costs include all of the following *except*:
    a. clinical supplies
    b. equipment costs
    c. depreciation
    d. laboratory procedures

14. The accounts receivable trial balance:
    a. tells you how much the practice owes to creditors
    b. shows any problems between the daily journal and the ledger
    c. tracks all disbursements and compares the total with the purchases
    d. uses an NCR transfer strip to copy pertinent information

15. Calculating and reviewing costs provide ambulatory care settings with:
    a. profit determining
    b. practice performance monitoring
    c. off-line batch processing
    d. a and b

CERTIFICATION REVIEW

These questions are designed to mimic the certification examinations. You can use these questions like a small "Certification Examination Study Guide," but this is not meant to take the place of the more extensive study guides. Use this portion to determine in what areas to concentrate your efforts when studying for the certification examination.

1. For the sake of accounting, a liability is:
    a. the cost of doing business
    b. considered overhead
    c. an expense
    d. a credit
    e. all of the above

2. Of the following statements, which is false?
    a. Double-entry bookkeeping is expensive.
    b. Double-entry bookkeeping is accurate.

   c. Double-entry bookkeeping is more time consuming.

   d. Double-entry bookkeeping has checks and balances in place.

3. Owner's equity is not the same as:
   a. net worth
   b. proprietorship
   c. capital
   d. accounts payable

4. Bonds may be purchased to do the following:
   a. protect the practice from embezzlement
   b. protect the practice from financial loss
   c. protect the practice from malpractice suits
   d. a and b
   e. all of the above

CASE STUDY

When the offices of Drs. Lewis and King agreed to accept individuals covered by a large managed care organization, the decision of the physician–owners was based on a complete financial analysis and projection of the expected effects the new patient load would have on the medical practice. As a result, the group practice added a second office manager and a new clinical medical assistant to the existing staff.

Discuss the following:
1. As Drs. Lewis and King absorb the new managed care patients into the practice, what can the physician–owners do to determine whether their financial analysis and projection was accurate?
2. Once the practice has assembled financial data on the effects of the new patient load, how will these data be used?
3. What beneficial effects might the addition of a clinical medical assistant have on the medical practice?

SELF-ASSESSMENT

Personal finances, as well as the finances of businesses such as ambulatory care settings, require careful planning, management, and budgeting. You can use the systems of business financial management to gain insights into your personal spending patterns and to help develop and fine-tune smart financial habits and attitudes.

For each statement, circle the response that best describes you.

1. I think saving money is:
   a. Important; I make every effort to put away a sum of money as savings on a regular basis.
   b. Great if you can find a way; I'd like to save, but I have trouble finding ways to do it.
   c. Not important right now; I have too many expenses—what I really need is a loan!

2. When planning a large purchase, such as a computer or a car, I:
   a. set a limit for spending and affordable installment payments and stick to it
   b. have a rough idea of what I can afford, but do not do any advance planning
   c. try to buy what I want and think about paying for it later

3. When considering monthly personal income and expenses, I:
   a. know exactly how much money is coming in and how much is going out to pay bills
   b. know I can cover my bills but do not keep track of exactly how much I make or spend
   c. hope for the best and if I fall short—charge it!

4. When I have extra money, I:
   a. save one third, use one third to pay off debts, and use the last third on a special purchase
   b. save half or use it to pay off debts and spend the other half on a special purchase
   c. spend it all on a special purchase

5. My checkbook is:
   a. always balanced
   b. sometimes balanced
   c. rarely balanced

6. When choosing a bank for my savings or checking, I:
   a. research interest rates, features, funds, and services carefully to find the best deal
   b. choose the bank that pays the highest interest rate
   c. just pick whatever is most convenient; banks are all the same

7. I think planning for retirement is:
   a. a priority now; the sooner you start saving, the more your money grows!
   b. important but not the most essential financial responsibility I have right now.
   c. not something I think about now—that's too far away; who can predict the future?

8. People think of me as:
   a. someone who pays attention to detail and is neat and organized
   b. someone who always manages to get the job done at the last minute
   c. someone who struggles to keep up with routine or repetitive tasks

9. I think analyzing financial data is:
   a. a smart way to assess current spending patterns and guide future spending
   b. a great thing to do if you have enough time and willpower
   c. a waste of time; besides, I just don't want to know

10. I am the kind of person who:

   a. sets short- and long-term financial goals for income and spending and works toward implementing them in a responsible way

   b. has short- and long-term financial goals but can not get around to planning for them

   c. makes financial decisions on a day-to-day basis; it is enough to deal with one day at a time

Scoring: If your answers were mostly A responses, congratulations! You have developed a financially responsible outlook and good recordkeeping habits. If your responses were mostly *B*s, you are thinking about financial realities and recognize the importance of a strong financial awareness. Focus on specific areas where you can improve your financial skills. If your responses were mostly *C*s, you need to work on achieving good personal financial habits. Start working on your recordkeeping skills by taking the plunge and keeping a weekly journal of expenses to see where your money goes!

CHAPTER POST-TEST

This is similar to the Pre-Test. Perform this test without looking at the book. This is just to see how well you have understood and can recall the information presented in this chapter after you have studied it and completed the workbook exercises. You will not be graded on this portion (other than the grade you give yourself), but this is an excellent preparation for your instructor's test. You may use this Post-Test to determine what areas you need to study more. Justify any "false" answers.

1. Accounts payable is the amount the physician is owed by patients. (T or F)

2. The purpose of cost analysis is to:

   a. determine the costs of each service

   b. determine the fixed costs

   c. determine the variable costs

   d. determine the total of all of the above

3. Both profits and expenses should be shown on income statements. (T or F)

4. Employees withholding allowance is recorded on the W-4 Form. (T or F)

CERTIFICATION CRITERIA CHECKLIST

As you go through your education and training, keep in mind the national certification examination that you will take when you graduate. Each chapter of the textbook and workbook covers a different section of the examination criteria. To keep track of your preparation for the certification examination turn to the back of this workbook and highlight the following CMA, RMA, or CMAS certification examination criteria (if you have already highlighted them from a previous chapter, put a check mark by the criteria):

CMA
I.   Computer Concepts
       3.   Computer applications
Q.   Managing Practice Finances
       1.   Bookkeeping systems
       4.   Accounting and banking procedures
       5.   Employee payroll

RMA
II.   Administrative Medical Assisting
       B.   Finance/Bookkeeping

CMAS
6. Medical Office Financial Management
- Fundamentals of financial management
- Patient accounts

COMPETENCY ASSESSMENT

Procedure 21-1 Preparing Accounts Receivable Trial Balance

Performance Objectives: A trial balance will determine if there is any problem between the daily journal and the ledger or patient accounts. Perform this objective within 20 minutes with a minimum score of 50 points.

Supplies/Equipment: Patient accounts, calculator, computer and software for computerized systems

Charting/Documentation: Enter appropriate documentation/charting in the box.

_____

_____

_____

_____

Instructor's/Evaluator's Comments and Suggestions:

_____

_____

_____

_____

_____

_____

SKILLS CHECKLIST Procedure 21-1: Preparing Accounts Receivable Trial Balance

Name _____

Date _____

No.	Skill	Check #1 20 pts ea	Check #2 10 pts ea	Check #3 5 pts ea	Notes
1	Pull all patient accounts that have a balance due.				
2	Enter the balance of those accounts into the calculator.				
3	Add the balances and total.				
4	Create an accounts receivable total.				
	a. Enter the accounts receivable total for the month.				
	b. Add total charges for the month. Subtotal.				
	c. Total the amount of payments received for the month.				
	d. Subtract the total payments from the total of "b" above. Subtotal.				
	e. Total the amount of the month's adjustments from the subtotal of "d" above.				
	f. Record the accounts receivable amount.				
Student's Total Points					
Points Possible (10 steps)		200	100	50	
Final Score (Student's Total Points / Possible Points)					

	Notes
Start time:	
End time:	
Total time: (20 min goal)	

EVALUATION OF CHAPTER KNOWLEDGE

Skills	Student Self-Evaluation		
	Good	Average	Poor
I know the importance of medical financial management in the ambulatory care setting.	_____	_____	_____
I understand and can define basic accounting terms.	_____	_____	_____
I can identify and have a working knowledge of the various accounting and bookkeeping systems.	_____	_____	_____
I understand the role computerized systems can play in the medical office.	_____	_____	_____
I recognize the challenges of converting from a manual to a computerized accounting system.	_____	_____	_____
I possess a working knowledge of cost analysis, financial records, and financial ratios.	_____	_____	_____
I understand utilization review and the importance it has in the ambulatory care setting.	_____	_____	_____
I recognize the importance of good personal and professional financial practices and habits.	_____	_____	_____

CHAPTER 22

The Medical Assistant as Office Manager

CHAPTER PRE-TEST

Perform this test without looking at the book. This is just to see how well you have understood and can recall the information in this chapter after you have read it, but before you have completed the workbook exercises. You will not be graded on this portion (other than the grade you give yourself). Justify any "false" answers.

1. Teamwork results in getting more accomplished with the resources available. (T or F)

2. Office managers do not need effective communication skills. (T or F)

3. It is not necessary to update the office procedures manual. (T or F)

4. Minutes should be sent only to the team members who attended the meeting. (T or F)

5. When working with an externing student, each step should be explained together with the rationale. (T or F)

6. Office managers need to be able to accept and offer criticism constructively. (T or F)

7. The person who is the office manager is also the human resources manager. (T or F)

INTRODUCTION

In the ambulatory care setting, the office manager is an important and essential staff member involved in the daily operation of the practice. The office manager is responsible for a wide variety of duties, including supervision, time management, finances, purchasing, marketing, education, and personnel. In some cases, the same individual serves as both the office manager and the human resources manager. With more facilities turning to managed care as a way to ensure consumer use of the appropriate level of care and to facilitate cost containment, opportunities exist for medical assistants to advance to the office manager position. Use this workbook chapter to explore the role of the office manager in the ambulatory care setting.

PERFORMANCE OBJECTIVES

After successful completion of this chapter you will be able to explain the medical terms related to managing a medical office. You will become familiar with the qualities a good manager and leader should possess and cultivate; you will recognize different management styles and will be able to determine which might be more effective in a given situation. You will be more aware of effective teamwork and how to properly coordinate and run meetings. You will have tools to increase productivity and effectively manage time. You will be able to describe the concepts of marketing and recall effective marketing tools, as well as how to create patient brochures and information flyers. You will have an understanding of payroll processing, employee benefits, taxes, financial management, risk management, liability coverage, and bonding. *The following statements are related to your learning objectives for this chapter. Fill in the blanks in the following paragraph with the appropriate term(s).*

The position of office manager may include the duties of (1) _____ _____ person. Good managers are also good (2) _____ and possesses many qualities. They provide their coworkers with (3) _____, (4) _____, and a feeling of ownership in the process. They manage to accomplish things without (5) _____, usually by the power of their personal (6) _____. It is also important that managers (7) _____ convey their (8) _____ to their employees. A source of ill feelings is often the (9) _____ to let employees know what is (10) _____ of them. Among the specific traits a manager should possess are effective (11) _____ skills, (12) _____, (13) _____, (14) _____ skills, (15) _____, (16) _____ skills, (17) _____ expertise, and (18) _____. A good manager is continually (19) _____. People who succeed will take responsibility for their (20) _____. People who do not manage well will (21) _____ others for their failures. Mindsets can be changed by coming to terms with what you have to (22) _____, (23) _____ what you really want to (24) _____, put your goals in writing using (25) _____ terms, begin with small (26) _____ goals, (27) _____ poor work habits such as (28) _____ _____, and tune out (29) _____ thoughts while focusing on positive thoughts. Office managers must wear many hats. They will often serve as a Security Officer. The responsibilities of the (30) _____ include (31) _____ and (32) _____ the various impacts of (33) _____ on each department and assisting with (34) _____ issues related to Health Insurance Portability and Accountability Act (HIPAA) regulations. There are two basic management styles: (35) _____ style and (36) _____ style. A technique used by managers to stay informed and connected with the health of the office is called MBWA or (37) _____. The office manager should (38) _____ a (39) _____ management procedure that assesses the risks to which he or she and the (40) _____ are exposed and takes steps to develop (41) _____ that (42) _____ those risks. Some common risks are: loss of a (43) _____ employee, failure of a (44) _____ or contractor, (45) _____ disclosure of (46) _____ information through error or (47) _____ entry, (48) _____ failure, (49) _____ to a staff member or nonemployee, and a personal (50) _____ change. New personnel orientation consists of (51) _____ and training new employees in the medical protocols and procedures (52) _____ to that practice. If the (53) _____ manual is detailed and accurate, the manual becomes a (54) _____ for the new employee. Assigning a (55) _____ who can respond to questions is also important. Most new employees will be on (56) _____ for (57) _____. Supervising student (58) _____ is another important part of medical office management, although the direct supervision can be (59) _____ to another supervisor who will work more directly with the student. Performance evaluations and salary reviews should be done on a (60) _____ basis that is predetermined by office policy. Conflict resolution is a skill that managers need to become (61) _____ at. There are many guidelines that are helpful in (62) _____ and (63) _____ conflict. Dismissing employees is another duty of the office manager. In this case, the written (64) _____ actually provides the format for the dismissal when necessary.

VOCABULARY BUILDER

Find the words listed below that are misspelled; circle them, and then correctly spell them in the spaces provided. Then insert the correct vocabulary terms into the sentences that follow.

agenda	"going bare"	practicum
ancilliary services	liability	procedures manual
benchmarking	malpractice	professional liability insurance
benefits	marketing	risk management
bond	minutes	teamwork
embezzle	negligance	work statement
externs		
	_____	_____

1. _____ refers to professional occupational companies hired to complete a specific job.

2. Legal responsibility is commonly referred to as _____.

3. _____ describes the situation of a physician who does not carry professional liability insurance.

4. Making a comparison between different organizations relative to how they accomplish tasks, remunerate employees, and so on is called _____.

5. _____ is designed to protect assets in the event a liability claim is filed and awarded.

6. _____ are a written record of topics discussed and actions taken during meeting sessions.

7. A _____ provides a concise description of the work you plan to accomplish.

8. A _____ is a binding agreement with an employee ensuring recovery of financial loss should funds be stolen or embezzled.

9. A printed list of topics to be discussed during a meeting is called an _____.

10. _____ is the process by which the provider of services makes the consumer aware of the scope and quality of those services. Examples might include public relations, brochures, patient education seminars, and newsletters.

11. _____ involves persons synergistically working together.

12. The failure to perform an act that a reasonable and prudent physician would or would not perform is _____.

13. The student _____ is a transitional stage providing an opportunity to apply theory learned in the classroom to a health care setting through practical, hands-on experience.

14. Remuneration that is in addition to the salary is a _____.

15. The office manager should schedule an informational interview with the _____ student before the practicum begins.

16. To appropriate fraudulently for one's own use is to _____.

17. _____ involves the identification, analysis, and treatment of risks within the medical office or facility.

18. The _____ provides detailed information relative to the performance of tasks within the job description.

19. _____ is the term commonly used today to describe professional liability.

LEARNING REVIEW

1. The office manager of a medical office or ambulatory care facility can have many varied responsibilities based on individual facility needs. What are five duties that are the responsibility of the office manager in a health care setting?

    (1) _____

    (2) _____

    (3) _____

    (4) _____

    (5) _____

2. Most marketing tools used in a medical environment provide educational and office services information to patients, potential patients, and the local community. Match the following marketing tools with their potential use in the ambulatory care facility setting.

    A. Seminars

    B. Brochures

    C. Newsletters

    D. Press releases

    E. Special events

    1. _____ These are used for announcing new equipment, new staff, expanded or remodeled office space, and so on.

    2. _____ These typically come in two types—patient education and office services—and present a professional image of the ambulatory care setting.

    3. _____ These provide an effective way to join with other community organizations to promote wellness.

    4. _____ These can educate patients and provide good will in the community. All facility staff can work as a team to organize these.

    5. _____ These can include a wide range of information from health-related topics to staff introductions to insurance updates. They may form the nucleus of a marketing program.

3. What are five attributes needed to perform as a quality manager in any office setting?

    (1) _____   (4) _____

    (2) _____   (5) _____

    (3) _____

CERTIFICATION REVIEW

These questions are designed to mimic the certification examinations. You can use these questions like a small "Certification Examination Study Guide," but this is not meant to take the place of the more extensive study guides. Use this portion to determine in what areas to concentrate your efforts when studying for the certification examination.

1. There is a direct correlation between a person's management style and his or her:
   a. technical expertise
   b. educational level
   c. personality
   d. salary

2. When managers delegate as much responsibility as possible to those they supervise, it is called:
   a. management by style
   b. management by exception
   c. management by decision model
   d. management by competitive edge

3. The person who applies the team-oriented management style is often comfortable with:
   a. teaching and coaching
   b. building, constructing, and modeling
   c. ideas, information, and data
   d. all of the above

4. A comprehensive safety program is essential to:
   a. marketing functions
   b. team building
   c. risk management
   d. equipment and supply maintenance

5. Leadership for the twenty-first century includes components of flexibility, mentoring, and:
   a. networking
   b. domination
   c. hierarchy
   d. rigidity

CASE STUDY

Office manager Shirley Brooks is responsible for the preparation and distribution of payroll checks at the offices of Drs. Lewis and King. Because the group practice is in the process of upgrading the computer system to accommodate a recent influx of new patients, Shirley is temporarily preparing the payroll using the manual write-it-once bookkeeping system. She is careful to consult payroll records for each employee, which include the employee's name, address, and telephone number; Social Security number; number of exemptions claimed on the W-4 form; gross salary; deductions withheld for all taxes, including Social Security, federal, state, local, unemployment, and disability; and date of employment.

Discuss the following:
1. As Shirley writes out the payroll check for Audrey Jones, CMA, what information should be included on the paycheck stub?
2. What must the physician's office have to process payroll?
3. What responsibility does the office manager have with regard to the confidentiality of payroll records? How might employees' rights to privacy be maintained?

SELF-ASSESSMENT

Put yourself in the place of the office manager.

1. What type of management style do you think you are the most comfortable with?

2. Carefully read about each type of style and explain why you think you are that type.

3. What skills will come naturally to you?

4. What skills will you have to work on the most?

POST-TEST

This is similar to the Pre-Test. Perform this test without looking at the book. This is just to see how well you have understood and can recall the information presented in this chapter after you have studied it and completed the workbook exercises. You will not be graded on this portion (other than the grade you give yourself), but this is an excellent preparation for your instructor's test. You may use this Post-Test to determine what areas you need to study more. Justify any "false" answers.

1. Teamwork results in getting less accomplished with the resources available. (T or F)

2. Office managers need effective communication skills. (T or F)

3. It is necessary to update the office procedures manual. (T or F)

4. Minutes should be sent all team members, not just those who attended the meeting. (T or F)

5. When working with an externing student, each step does not need to be explained together with the rationale, because they already have training. (T or F)

6. Office managers need to be able to offer criticism constructively, but they should not have to accept criticism. (T or F)

7. The person who is the office manager is never the human resources manager. (T or F)

CERTIFICATION CRITERIA CHECKLIST

As you go through your education and training, keep in mind the national certification examination that you will take when you graduate. Each chapter of the textbook and workbook covers a different section of the examination criteria. To keep track of your preparation for the certification examination, turn to the back of this workbook and highlight the following CMA, RMA, or CMAS certification examination criteria (if you have already highlighted them from a previous chapter, put a check mark by the criteria):

CMA

C. Psychology
    1. Basic principles
D. Professionalism
    5. Working as a team member to achieve goals
E. Communication
    5. Evaluating and understanding communication
F. Medicolegal Guidelines & Requirements
M. Resource Information and Community Services
N. Managing Physician's Professional Schedule and Travel
O. Managing the Office
P. Office Policies and Procedures
Q. Managing Practice Finances
    5. Employee payroll

RMA

I. General Medical Assisting Knowledge
    C. Medical Law
    D. Medical Ethics
    E. Human Relations
    F. Patient Education
        2. Patient resource materials

CMAS

1. Medical Assisting Foundation
   - Legal and ethical considerations
   - Professionalism
3. Medical Office Clerical Assisting
   - Patient information and community resources
4. Medical Records Management
6. Medical Office Financial Management
8. Medical Office Management

COMPETENCY ASSESSMENT

Procedure 22-1 Preparing a Meeting Agenda

Performance Objectives: To prepare a meeting agenda with an established list of specific items to be discussed or acted on, or both. Perform this objective within 20 minutes with a minimum score of 30 points.

Supplies/Equipment: List of participants, the order of business, names of individuals giving reports, names of any guest speakers, a computer, paper to print agendas on

Charting/Documentation: Enter appropriate documentation/charting in the box.

_____

_____

_____

_____

Instructor's/Evaluator's Comments and Suggestions:

_____

_____

_____

_____

_____

_____

SKILLS CHECKLIST Procedure 22-1: Preparing a Meeting Agenda

Name _____

Date _____

No.	Skill	Check #1 20 pts ea	Check #2 10 pts ea	Check #3 5 pts ea	Notes
1	Confirm the proposed dates and place of meeting.				
2	Collect information from previous meetings' minutes for old agenda items. Check with others for report items and determine any new business.				
3	Prepare the meeting agenda and have it approved by the meeting chair.				
4	Send agenda to participants 2 weeks in advance.				
5	Reserve the meeting room.				
6	Schedule food items, equipment, and supplies that may be needed.				
Student's Total Points					
Points Possible		120	60	30	
Final Score (Student's Total Points / Possible Points)					

	Notes
Start time:	
End time:	
Total time: (20 min goal)	

COMPETENCY ASSESSMENT

Procedure 22-2 Supervising a Student Practicum

Performance Objectives: To prepare a training path for a student extern being assigned to the office, make the involved personnel aware of their responsibilities, preplan the jobs the student will perform and in what sequence they will be assigned, and try to make the externship successful by providing as much supervision and assistance as necessary. Perform this objective within 30 minutes with a minimum score of 55 points.

Supplies/Equipment: A schedule log, calendar, office procedures manual, any criteria presented by the program director

Charting/Documentation: Enter appropriate documentation/charting in the box.

_____

_____

_____

_____

Instructor's/Evaluator's Comments and Suggestions:

_____

_____

_____

_____

_____

SKILLS CHECKLIST Procedure 22-2: Supervising a Student Practicum

Name _____

Date _____

No.	Skill	Check #1 20 pts ea	Check #2 10 pts ea	Check #3 5 pts ea	Notes
1	Determine the amount of supervision the student will require.				
2	Indentify the supervisor who will be immediately responsible for the extern.				
3	Follow Web page instructions for making arrangements.				
4	Plan which tasks the extern will be perfoming.				
5	Create a schedule outlining the time the student will be assigned to each unit/area.				
6	Begin orientation for the extern as soon as he or she arrives. Include a tour of the office and an introduction to the staff.				
7	Maintain an accurate record of the hours the extern works. Log the dates and reasons for any missed days, late arrivals, or early dismissals.				
8	Check with the extern frequently to be sure the student is receiving meaningful training from the work experience.				
9	Consult with the physicians and staff members with whom the student has worked for their opinion of the student's capabilities. Follow up with any problems that might be identified.				
10	Report the extern's progress to the medical assisting program director either during an on-site visit or via phone/e-mail.				
11	Prepare the student's evaluation report from input from all who worked with the student.				
Student's Total Points					
Points Possible		220	110	55	
Final Score (Student's Total Points / Possible Points)					

	Notes
Start time:	
End time:	
Total time: (30 min goal, including meeting with director, setting schedule, etc.)	

COMPETENCY ASSESSMENT

Procedure 22-3 Making Travel Arrangements

Performance Objectives: To make travel arrangements for the physician. Perform this objective within 20 minutes with a minimum score of 30 points.

Supplies/Equipment: A travel plan/preferences, telephone, directory, computer, and the physician's or office credit card to secure reservations

Charting/Documentation: Enter appropriate documentation/charting in the box.

_____

_____

_____

_____

Instructor's/Evaluator's Comments and Suggestions:

_____

_____

_____

_____

_____

_____

SKILLS CHECKLIST Procedure 22-3: Making Travel Arrangements

Name _____

Date _____

No.	Skill	Check #1 20 pts ea	Check #2 10 pts ea	Check #3 5 pts ea	Notes
1	Confirm the details of the trip: dates, times, places of departures and arrivals, preferred transportation method, number of travelers, preferred lodging type and price range, and if traveler's checks will be required.				
2	Telephone travel agent or use online ticket services.				
3	Pick up tickets, arrange for delivery, or secure confirmation of electronic tickets.				
4	Checks that arrangements are accurate and confirmed.				
5	Check that car rental and room reservations are accurate and confirmed.				
6	Make additional copies of the itinerary or create the itinerary: list dates and times of arrivals and departures, including flight numbers and seat assignments; modes of transportation; names, addresses, phone numbers, and e-mail addresses of hotels and meeting places. Maintain a copy for the office. Forward several copies to the physician.				
Student's Total Points					
Points Possible		120	60	30	
Final Score (Student's Total Points / Possible Points)					

	Notes
Start time:	
End time:	
Total time: (20 min goal)	

COMPETENCY ASSESSMENT

Procedure 22-4 Making Travel Arrangements via the Internet

Performance Objectives: To make travel arrangements for the physician using the Internet. Perform this objective within 20 minutes with a minimum score of 35 points.

Supplies/Equipment: A travel plan/preferences, computer, physician's or office credit card to secure reservations

Charting/Documentation: Enter appropriate documentation/charting in the box.

_____

_____

_____

_____

Instructor's/Evaluator's Comments and Suggestions:

_____

_____

_____

_____

_____

_____

SKILLS CHECKLIST Procedure 22-4: Making Travel Arrangements via the Internet

Name _____

Date _____

No.	Skill	Check #1 20 pts ea	Check #2 10 pts ea	Check #3 5 pts ea	Notes
1	Confirm the details of the trip: dates, times, places of departures and arrivals, preferred transportation method, number of travelers, preferred lodging type and price range, and if traveler's checks will be required.				
2	Access the Internet; select a search engine and locate Web pages under air fares with links to car rentals and hotels.				
3	Follow Web page instructions for making arrangements.				
4	Review and copy confirmations of transactions.				
5	Confirm how tickets will arrive, that is, picked up or electronic.				
6	Make additional copies of the itinerary for the office.				
7	Forward several copies to the physician.				
Student's Total Points					
Points Possible		140	70	35	
Final Score (Student's Total Points / Possible Points)					

	Notes
Start time:	
End time:	
Total time: (20 min goal)	

COMPETENCY ASSESSMENT

Procedure 22-5 Developing and Maintaining a Procedure Manual

Performance Objectives: To develop and maintain a comprehensive, up-to-date procedures manual covering each medical, technical, and administrative procedure in the office with step-by-step directions and rationale for performing each task. Perform this objective (one procedure) within 20 minutes with a minimum score of 45 points.

Supplies/Equipment: A computer, three-ring binder, paper, procedures and criteria

Charting/Documentation: Enter appropriate documentation/charting in the box.

_____

_____

_____

_____

Instructor's/Evaluator's Comments and Suggestions:

_____

_____

_____

_____

_____

_____

SKILLS CHECKLIST Procedure 22-5: Developing and Maintaining a Procedure Manual

Name _____

Date _____

No.	Skill	Check #1 20 pts ea	Check #2 10 pts ea	Check #3 5 pts ea	Notes
1	Write detailed step-by-step procedures and rationale for each medical, technical, and administrative function. Each procedure is written by experienced employees close to the function and reviewed by a supervisor or the office manager.				
2	Include regular maintenance (cleaning, servicing, and cali-brating) instructions and flow sheets for all office equipment, both in the clinical area and in the office/business areas.				
3	Include step-by-step procedures on how to accomplish each task both in the clinical area and in the office/business areas.				
4	Include local and out of the area resources for clinical staff, office/business staff, physicians/providers, and patients. Provide a listing in each area with contact information and services provided.				
5	Include basic rules and regula-tions, state and federal, which are related to processes performed in both clinical and office/business areas.				
6	Include the clinic procedures and flow sheets for taking inventory in each of the areas and instructions on ordering procedures.				
7	Collect the procedures into the office procedures manual.				

No.	Skill	Check #1 20 pts ea	Check #2 10 pts ea	Check #3 5 pts ea	Notes
8	Store one complete manual in a common library area. One complete copy goes to the physician–employer, to the office manager, and to each department.				
9	Review the manual annually; add any new procedures and delete and modify as needed.				
Student's Total Points					
Points Possible		180	90	45	
Final Score (Student's Total Points / Possible Points)					

	Notes
Start time:	
End time:	
Total time: (20 min goal)	

EVALUATION OF CHAPTER KNOWLEDGE

Skills	Student Self-Evaluation		
	Good	Average	Poor
I understand payroll processing and other employee-related financial duties, including computing taxes.	____	____	____
I exercise efficient time management techniques.	____	____	____
I understand risk management issues.	____	____	____
I understand the importance of developing and maintaining policy and procedures manuals.	____	____	____
I understand methods of public relations for the ambulatory care setting.	____	____	____
I can describe liability coverage and bonding.	____	____	____
I can describe the qualities of an effective office manager.	____	____	____
I am able to describe the process of supervising a student practicum.	____	____	____
I understand the importance of teamwork and its role when supervising personnel.	____	____	____

CHAPTER 23

The Medical Assistant as Human Resources Manager

CHAPTER PRE-TEST

Perform this test without looking at the book. This is just to see how well you have understood and can recall the information in this chapter after you have read it, but before you have completed the workbook exercises. You will not be graded on this portion (other than the grade you give yourself). Justify any "false" answers.

1. Which of the following is *not* a function of the human resources (HR) manager?
    a. creating and updating a policy manual
    b. recruiting and hiring office personnel
    c. orienting new personnel
    d. training new personnel

2. Wage and salary policies should be in writing. (T or F)

3. A policy manual should contain daily step-by-step instructions. (T or F)

4. Job descriptions are not always useful because they change so often. (T or F)

5. All job applicants should be interviewed. (T or F)

6. It is acceptable to ask job applicants about the last place they worked and a conflict they had there. (T or F)

7. References are usually checked upon after the first interview. (T or F)

8. The HR manager is responsible for dismissing employees. (T or F)

9. Employees have a right to review their personnel files at any time. (T or F)

INTRODUCTION

In some health care practices, particularly in that of the solo practitioner, the office manager also functions as the HR manager. In other cases, these management functions are assumed by two separate individuals. The HR manager is concerned with both group and individual employee issues. The HR manager performs such duties as formulating job descriptions, recruitment and hiring, payroll and salary review, training, benefits, advancement, grievances, dismissals, and maintaining employee personnel records. Use this workbook chapter to explore the role of the HR manager in the ambulatory care setting.

PERFORMANCE OBJECTIVES

After successful completion of this chapter you will be able to explain the medical terms related to HR management. You will be familiar with the duties of an HR manager; the functions of formal policies and the policy manual; and the methods and rules surrounding the recruitment, interviewing, and orienting of new employees. You will also know about the laws surrounding personnel issues and management. You will be aware of the reasons and purposes of exit interviews and maintaining accurate personnel records. *The following statements are related to your learning objectives for this chapter. Fill in the blanks in the following paragraph with the appropriate term(s).*

Tasks usually assigned to the HR manager include determining job (1) _____;

scheduling, hiring, and (2) _____ new employees; and (3) _____

employee personnel (4) _____. One difference between a procedures manual

and a policy manual is that the procedures manual is a daily, step-by-step guide with instructions,

whereas a policy manual is about (5) _____ practices and (6) _____

of an office. The HR manager also needs to make sure (7) _____ are

in place for every position. Included in the job description are the (8) _____

of the ideal applicant; the necessary (9) _____, (10) _____,

(11) _____; and any special (12) _____ or licensure

that is expected. The job description should be reviewed and updated every (13) _____.

A major challenge of HR managers today is that of (14) _____. Medical

assistants are listed as the number one fastest growing occupation through 2012 by the

(15) _____. The need is so great that

some clinics have turned to contracting out such work as (16) _____ and

(17) _____. Before interviews, it is a good idea to establish a set of

(18) _____ for the (19) _____. This helps alleviate

one applicant being given (20) _____ over another. At the close of the inter-

view, the applicant should be told when the (21) _____ will be made or whether a

(22) _____ will be conducted, as well as how (23) _____

will be made. At the time the offer for hire is made, the candidate should understand the

(24) _____ offered, the (25) _____, the practice

(26) _____, and the (27) _____. When the candidate accepts the

position, a (28) _____ letter should be written with further details. Orienting the new employee is the responsibility of both the (29) _____ and lead personnel. Training is usually the responsibility of the office manager and the staff supervisors where the new employee will be working. Important elements of orientation include (30) _____ to other (31) _____ members and (32) _____ a mentor. Dismissing employees usually falls to the (33) _____ with the HR manager involved in the exit interview. An important aspect of the HR manager is to maintain (34) _____. This confidential employee file should include all documentation and correspondence related to each employee from (35) _____ to (36) _____, from (37) _____ to (38) _____ including the formal (39) _____ and all demographic information. These files are kept for (40) _____ after the employee leaves the practice. HR managers must always comply with (41) _____ laws against (42) _____ on the basis of race, color, religion, sex, age, or national origin.

VOCABULARY BUILDER

Find the words listed below that are misspelled; circle them, and then correctly spell them in the spaces provided. Insert the correct vocabulary terms into the following sentences.

conflict resolution	job description	overtime
educational history	letter of referance	probation
evaluation	letter of resignation	résumés
exit interveiw	menter	salary review
involuntary dismisal	networking	work history

_____ _____ _____

_____

1. Clinical medical assistant Anna Preciado, who is approaching 1 year of employment at the offices of Drs. Lewis and King, is due to have her _____ to assess her job performance.

2. Because of an unexpected staffing shortfall, Audrey Jones, CMA, has volunteered to work _____ this week. She will receive 1½ times the regular rate of pay for hours above her regular 40-hour week.

3. Office manager Marilyn Johnson, acting as the HR manager, will conduct a _____ _____ at the beginning of the new calendar year with each employee. If necessary, she will then inform the employee of his or her revised base pay rate.

4. An _____ has been scheduled for administrative/clinical medical assistant Liz Corbin before she leaves the clinic to continue her education. This session will give Liz an opportunity to provide her positive and negative opinions of the position and the facility.

5. Jane O'Hara, co-office manager at Inner City Health Care, has been asked by her physician–employers to use _____ to solve several problems occurring between two coworkers at the facility.

6. Office manager Marilyn Johnson has received a _____ from the former instructor of a current job applicant describing the applicant's performance, attitude, and qualifications.

7. In interviews for a new Certified Medical Assistant position, office manager Walter Seals asks applicants to outline their _____, including employers, positions, duties, and responsibilities.

8. Office manager Walter Seals reviews _____ received from applicants for the new medical assisting position to ensure that the applicants interviewed meet the physician–employer's minimum qualifications for education and work experience.

9. The _____ listed on each résumé reveals to the office manager the applicant's places of learning and degrees or certificates earned.

10. The violation of office policies at Inner City Health Care led to the _____ of one of the part-time employees.

11. Administrative medical assistant Ellen Armstrong, in her first job since leaving school, has had office manager Marilyn Johnson as her _____, to assist in the training, guidance, and coaching she will need in her first position.

12. Winston Lewis, MD, is active in his state medical society; the _____ has resulted in beneficial and long-lasting social, business, and professional relationships.

13. Liz Corbin, CMA, submitted a _____ to her current employer when she decided to leave her present position to return to school to pursue an advanced degree.

14. Office manager Marilyn Johnson will inform all of the job applicants that they will be on _____ for their first 3 months on the job. During this period, the employee and supervisory personnel can determine if the environment and the position are satisfactory for the employee.

15. Office manager Jane O'Hara, updating the employee manual, includes a _____ for every position in the office that details tasks, duties, and responsibilities.

LEARNING REVIEW

1. The manual that identifies clear guidelines and directions required of all employees is known as the policy manual. What are four topics that would be included in a policy manual regardless of the size of the practice identified in this chapter.

   (1) _____

   (2) _____

   (3) _____

   (4) _____

2. Office manager Marilyn Johnson has the responsibility of dismissing an employee for a serious violation of office policies. From the list below, select key points to keep in mind when dismissal is necessary by circling the letters of the statements that apply.

    A. Have employee pack his or her belongings from desk.

    B. The dismissal should be made in private.

    C. Take no longer than 20 minutes for the dismissal.

    D. Be direct, firm, and to the point in identifying reasons.

    E. Explain terms of dismissal (keys, clearing out area, final paperwork).

    F. Do not listen to the employee's opinion and emotions.

    G. If he or she insists, allow the employee to finish the work of the day.

    H. Do not engage in an in-depth discussion of performance.

3. The job description must have enough information to provide both the supervisor and the employee with a clear outline of what the job entails. Name four items that must be included in a job description.

    (1) _____   (3) _____

    (2) _____   (4) _____

4. The interview worksheet is an excellent tool to make certain that the interviews with each candidate are fair and equitable. Provide six items that should be included on any interview worksheet.

    (1) _____   (4) _____

    (2) _____   (5) _____

    (3) _____   (6) _____

CERTIFICATION REVIEW

These questions are designed to mimic the certification examinations. You can use thee questions like a small "Certification Examination Study Guide," but this is not meant to take the place of the more extensive study guides. Use this portion to determine in what areas to concentrate your efforts when studying for the certification examination.

1. A salary review is:

    a. usually conducted at the beginning of the new year

    b. virtually the same as the performance review

    c. conducted on the anniversary date of hire

    d. normally done every 3 years

2. Questions regarding drug use, arrest records, and medical history during an interview are:

    a. appropriate

    b. inappropriate

    c. illegal

    d. none of the above

3. Title VII of the Civil Rights Act addresses:

   a. overtime pay

   b. discrimination based on race, age, and sex

   c. hiring and firing practices

   d. sexual harassment

4. When a candidate accepts a position, the HR manager should write a letter outlining the specifics of the job. This letter is called:

   a. a confirmation letter

   b. a congratulatory letter

   c. a recommendation letter

   d. a reference letter

5. A person with AIDS who satisfies the necessary skills for a job and has the experience and education required will be protected from discrimination by:

   a. OSHA

   b. CLIA

   c. AAMA

   d. ADA

CASE STUDY

Since the offices of Drs. Lewis and King have expanded to cover a rapidly growing patient load, including the hiring of a co-office manager and a new clinical medical assistant, the work pace has been hectic, but challenging. At the suggestion of Dr. Lewis, the office managers decide to hold a staff meeting to talk about ways to keep the lines of communication open and process the many changes occurring at the growing medical practice. Marilyn Johnson and Shirley Brooks encourage staff to be vocal with their feedback, suggestions, and concerns.

Discuss the following:
1. What other techniques can the office managers use to prevent or solve conflicts in the workplace during this period of growth and transition?
2. Why is effective communication one of the most important goals of the HR manager?

SELF-ASSESSMENT

1. If you were put into the position of hiring a new employee, what attributes would you be looking for?

   a. Make a list of the technical skills your new employee would need.

   b. Make a list of the affective behavior skills your new employee would need, including a positive attitude, good work ethics, and so forth.

    c. Determine how you could measure the technical skills you listed.

    d. Determine how you could measure the softer skills of affective behavior you listed in item b above. How could you determine those qualities?

    e. Which is more difficult to measure: technical or behavioral? Which is more difficult to train?

2. When you interview for a job, what technical and behavioral skills on your lists will you need to improve on?

POST-TEST

This is similar to the Pre-Test. Perform this test without looking at the book. This is just to see how well you have understood and can recall the information presented in this chapter after you have studied it and completed the workbook exercises. You will not be graded on this portion (other than the grade you give yourself), but this is an excellent preparation for your instructor's test. You may use this Post-Test to determine what areas you need to study more. Justify any "false" answers.

1. Which of the following are functions of the HR manager? (circle all the apply)

    a. creating and updating a policy manual

    b. training new personnel

    c. recruiting and hiring office personnel

    d. orienting new personnel

2. Wage and salary policies need not be in writing as long as both parties agree. (T or F)

3. A policy manual should contain general policies and practices of the office. (T or F)

4. Job descriptions are always useful and should be clearly written. (T or F)

5. Only qualified job applicants should be interviewed. (T or F)

6. It is good to ask job applicants about conflicts they have had and how they solved them. (T or F)

7. References are usually checked before the first interview. (T or F)

8. The HR manager is responsible for the exit interview, but usually not for dismissing employees. (T or F)

9. Employees do not have the right to review their personnel files unless requested by an attorney. (T or F)

CERTIFICATION CRITERIA CHECKLIST

As you go through your education and training, keep in mind the national certification examination that you will take when you graduate. Each chapter of the textbook and workbook covers a different section of the examination criteria. To keep track of your preparation for the certification examination, turn to the back of this workbook and highlight the following CMA, RMA, or CMAS certification examination criteria (if you have already highlighted them from a previous chapter, put a check mark by the criteria):

CMA
C. Psychology
      1. Basic principles
E. Communication
      6. Interviewing techniques
F. Medicolegal Guidelines & Requirements
O. Managing the Office
      1. Maintaining the physical plant
P. Office Policies and Procedures

RMA
I. General Medical Assisting Knowledge
      C. Medical Law
      D. Medical Ethics
      E. Human Relations
      F. Patient Education
          2. Patient resource materials

CMAS
1. Medical Assisting Foundation
      • Legal and ethical considerations
      • Professionalism
8. Medical Office Management
      • Human resources

COMPETENCY ASSESSMENT

Procedure 23-1 Develop and Maintain a Policy Manual

Performance Objectives: To develop and maintain a comprehensive, up-to-date policy manual of all office policies relating to employee practices, benefits, office conduct, and so forth. Perform this objective within 20 minutes (for one policy) with a minimum score of 35 points.

Supplies/Equipment: Computer, three-ring binder, paper, standard policy format

Charting/Documentation: Enter appropriate documentation/charting in the box.

_____

_____

_____

_____

Instructor's/Evaluator's Comments and Suggestions:

_____

_____

_____

_____

_____

_____

SKILLS CHECKLIST Procedure 23-1: Develop and Maintain a Policy Manual

Name _____

Date _____

No.	Skill	Check #1 20 pts ea	Check #2 10 pts ea	Check #3 5 pts ea	Notes
1	Following office format, develop precise, written office policies detailing all necessary information pertaining to the staff and their positions. Include benefits, vacation, sick leave, hours, dress codes, evaluations, rules of conduct, and grounds for dismissal.				
2	Identify procedures for reimbursing overtime, preventing discrimination and harassment, creating a safe workplace, and allowing for jury duty.				
3	Include a policy statement related to smoking and other substances.				
4	Identify steps to follow should an employee become disabled during employment.				
5	Determine what employee opportunities for continuing education will be reimbursed and include requirements for certification and licensures.				
6	Provide a copy of the policy manual for each employee.				
7	Review and update the policy manual regularly. Add or delete items as necessary, dating each revision.				
Student's Total Points					
Points Possible		140	70	35	
Final Score (Student's Total Points / Possible Points)					

	Notes
Start time:	
End time:	
Total time: (20 min goal for one policy)	

COMPETENCY ASSESSMENT
Procedure 23-2 Prepare a Job Description

Performance Objectives: To develop a precise definition of the tasks assigned to a job, to determine the expectations and level of competency required, and to specify the experience, training, and education needed to perform the job for purposes of recruiting and performance evaluation. Perform this objective within 20 minutes (for one job description) with a minimum score of 30 points.

Supplies/Equipment: Computer, three-ring binder, paper, standard job description format

Charting/Documentation: Enter appropriate documentation/charting in the box.

_____

_____

_____

_____

Instructor's/Evaluator's Comments and Suggestions:

_____

_____

_____

_____

_____

SKILLS CHECKLIST Procedure 23-2: Prepare a Job Description

Name _____

Date _____

No.	Skill	Check #1 20 pts ea	Check #2 10 pts ea	Check #3 5 pts ea	Notes
1	Detail each task that creates the job.				
2	List special medical, technical, or clerical skills needed.				
3	Determine the level of education, training, and experience required for the position.				
4	Determine where the job fits into the overall structure of the office.				
5	Specify any unusual working conditions (hours, locations, etc.) that may apply.				
6	Describe career path opportunities.				
Student's Total Points					
Points Possible		120	60	30	
Final Score (Student's Total Points / Possible Points)					

	Notes
Start time:	
End time:	
Total time: (20 min goal)	

COMPETENCY ASSESSMENT

Procedure 23-3 Conduct Interviews

Performance Objectives: To screen applicants for training, experience, and characteristics to select the best candidate to fill the position vacancy. Perform this objective within 40 minutes with a minimum score of 85 points.

Supplies/Equipment: Interview questions; policy manual (for referencing); applicant's résumé, application, and cover letter

Charting/Documentation: Enter appropriate documentation/charting in the box.

_____

_____

_____

_____

Instructor's/Evaluator's Comments and Suggestions:

_____

_____

_____

_____

_____

_____

SKILLS CHECKLIST Procedure 23-3: Conduct Interviews

Name _____

Date _____

No.	Skill	Check #1 20 pts ea	Check #2 10 pts ea	Check #3 5 pts ea	Notes
1	Review résumés and applications received.				
2	Select candidates who most closely match the education and experience being sought.				
3	Create an interview worksheet for each candidate, listing the points to cover.				
4	Select an interview team. Include the office manager and immediate supervisor of the position being filled.				
5	Call personally to schedule the interview. This will allow you to judge the applicant's telephone voice and manners.				
6	Remind the interviewers of the various legal restrictions concerning questions that can be asked.				
7	Conduct interviews in a quiet, private setting.				
8	Put the applicant at ease by beginning with an overview about the practice and staff, briefly describing the job and answering preliminary questions.				
9	Ask questions about the applicant's work experience and educational background using the résumé and interview worksheet as a guideline.				
10	Provide the most promising applicants additional information about the benefits and a tour of the office if practical.				
11	Applicant's general salary requirements may be discussed, but avoid discussion of a specific salary until a formal offer is tendered.				
12	Inform the applicants when a decision will be made, and thank each applicant for participating in the interview.				
13	Do not make a job offer until all the candidates have been interviewed.				

No.	Skill	Check #1 20 pts ea	Check #2 10 pts ea	Check #3 5 pts ea	Notes
14	Check references of all prospective employees.				
15	Establish a second interview between the physician–employer(s) and the qualified candidate if necessary.				
16	Confirm accepted job offers in writing, specifying the details of the offer and acceptance.				
17	Notify all unsuccessful applicants by letter when the position has been filled.				
Student's Total Points					
Points Possible		340	170	85	
Final Score (Student's Total Points / Possible Points)					

	Notes
Start time:	
End time:	
Total time: (40 min goal, includes preinterview meeting of committee and postinterview meeting)	

COMPETENCY ASSESSMENT

Procedure 23-4 Orient Personnel

Performance Objectives: To acquaint new employees with office policies, staff, what the job encompasses, procedures to be performed, and job performance expectations. Perform this objective within 30 minutes with a minimum score of 45 points.

Supplies/Equipment: Policy manual

Charting/Documentation: Enter appropriate documentation/charting in the box.

_____

_____

_____

_____

Instructor's/Evaluator's Comments and Suggestions:

_____

_____

_____

_____

_____

SKILLS CHECKLIST Procedure 23-4: Orient Personnel

Name _____

Date _____

No.	Skill	Check #1 20 pts ea	Check #2 10 pts ea	Check #3 5 pts ea	Notes
1	Tour the facilities and introduce the office staff.				
2	Complete employee-related documents and explain their purpose.				
3	Explain the benefits program.				
4	Present the office policy manual and discuss the key elements.				
5	Review federal and state regulatory precautions for medical facilities.				
6	Review the job description.				
7	Explain and demonstrate procedures to be performed and the use of procedures manuals supporting these procedures.				
8	Demonstrate the use of any specialized equipment (such as time clocks, key entries, etc.). Medical equipment will be demonstrated by clinical staff.				
9	Assign a mentor from the staff to help with the orientation.				
Student's Total Points					
Points Possible		180	90	45	
Final Score (Student's Total Points / Possible Points)					

	Notes
Start time:	
End time:	
Total time: (30 min goal)	

EVALUATION OF CHAPTER KNOWLEDGE

Skills	Student Self-Evaluation		
	Good	Average	Poor
I can describe the role of the HR manager.	——	——	——
I can explain the function of the office policy manual.	——	——	——
I can identify methods of recruiting employees for a medical practice.	——	——	——
I am familiar with the interview process.	——	——	——
I can describe appropriate evaluation tools for employees.	——	——	——
I can recall dismissal procedures.	——	——	——
I can identify items in employee personnel files.	——	——	——
I can define laws relating to personnel management.	——	——	——
I understand effective strategies for conflict resolution.	——	——	——

CHAPTER 24

Preparing for Medical Assisting Credentials

CHAPTER PRE-TEST

Perform this test without looking at the book. This is just to see how well you have understood and can recall the information in this chapter after you have read it, but before you have completed the workbook exercises. You will not be graded on this portion (other than the grade you give yourself). Justify any "false" answers.

1. A Registered Medical Assistant (RMA) and a Certified Medical Assistant (CMA) have the same bylaws and creed. (T or F)

2. A CMA may only work in the state in which the credentials were received. (T or F)

3. Three major areas included in the CMA examination are clinical, administrative, and general medical knowledge. (T or F)

4. Medical assistants may be trained on the job; however, physicians recognize that their offices operate much more efficiently and effectively with professionally trained and formally educated personnel. (T or F)

5. A CMA does not have to be a member of AAMA or currently employed to recertify. (T or F)

6. On meeting recertification requirements, the applicant will receive a new certificate. (T or F)

7. Once a student has become a member of AAMA, he or she may stay at the student rate for one year after graduation. (T or F)

INTRODUCTION

Certification provides established, consistent criteria for evaluating the professional competence of a medical assistant. The certification examination is offered by the American Association of Medical Assistants (AAMA). An individual who successfully passes the examination is awarded the Certified Medical Assistant (CMA) credential. In addition, the American Medical Technologists (AMT) organization conducts the examination that leads to the Registered Medical Assistant (RMA) credential. Certification is an important part of professional development and is highly valued by employers in the health care workplace. Use this workbook chapter to determine the specifics of the certification process.

PERFORMANCE OBJECTIVES

After successful completion of this chapter you will be able to explain the medical terms related to certification and recertification. You will be able to list the advantages and purposes of certification. You will be able to cite the professional organizations that sponsor the examinations and what credential is obtained by passing each examination. You will understand the requirement for recertification. *The following statements are related to your learning objectives for this chapter. Fill in the blanks in the following paragraph with the appropriate term(s).*

The CMA credential is awarded to those individuals who pass a national (1) _____ examination offered by the Certifying Board of the (2) _____ and administered by the (3) _____ (abbreviated NBME). The RMA credential is offered by the (4) _____. Only the (5) _____ examination requires formal education. The (6) _____ examination is available to persons with on-the-job experience. Both examinations require extensive knowledge in three basic areas: (7) _____, (8) _____, and (9) _____. (10) _____ of AAMA may take the certification examination at a reduced rate; students must enroll as members while they are still in school to take the examination at the (11) _____ rate. Once certified, the CMA must recertify every (12) _____ years. As of January 2005, CMAs are required to recertify by the (13) _____ of their birth month in the (14) _____ calendar year after certification/recertification. Recertification for the RMA credential requires an annual fee of (15) _____. The (16) _____ and the (17) _____ are national professional organizations that offer many benefits to their members.

VOCABULARY BUILDER

Match each correct vocabulary term to the aspect of the certification process that best describes it.

_____ 1. Certification Examination

_____ 2. Certified Medical Assistant (CMA)

_____ 3. Continuing Education Units (CEUs)

_____ 4. National Board of Medical Examiners (NBME)

_____ 5. Recertification

_____ 6. Registered Medical Assistant (RMA)

_____ 7. Task Force for Test Construction

A. Method for earning points toward recertification

B. A standardized means of evaluating medical assistant competency

C. Maintaining current CMA status

D. Credential awarded for successfully passing the Certification Examination

E. Committee of professionals whose responsibility is to update the CMA examination annually to reflect changes in medical assistants' responsibilities and to include new developments in medical knowledge and technology

F. Credential awarded for successfully passing the AMT Examination

G. Consultants for the Certification Examination

LEARNING REVIEW

1. The AAMA Certification Examination is a comprehensive test of the knowledge actually used in today's medical office. The test is updated annually to include the latest changes in medical assistants' daily responsibilities. In addition, the updates include the latest developments in medical knowledge and technology. Name the three major areas tested in the Certification Examination and describe what each includes.

    (1) _____

    (2) _____

    (3) _____

2. A. Health care professionals today should maintain a lifelong commitment to _____

    _____ .

    B. To keep their _____ current, CMAs are required to recertify

    every _____ .

    C. A total of _____ points is necessary to recertify the basic CMA credential.

    D. Continuing education courses are offered by _____

    groups.

3. A. What is the address, telephone number, and web address for obtaining an application for the Certification Examination (Choose either AAMA or AMT)?

    _____

    _____

    _____

    B. What guide for the Certification Examination is available from the AAMA?

    _____

    C. What program and what bimonthly publication does the AAMA make available to members who are interested in pursuing continuing education credits?

    Program: _____

    Publication: _____

CERTIFICATION REVIEW

These questions are designed to mimic the certification examinations. You can use these questions like a small "Certification Examination Study Guide," but this is not meant to take the place of the more extensive study guides. Use this portion to determine in what areas to concentrate your efforts when studying for the certification examination.

1. General medical assisting knowledge on the AMT Certification Examination includes anatomy and physiology, medical terminology, and:
   a. insurance and billing
   b. medical ethics
   c. bookkeeping and filing
   d. first aid

2. The organization that develops licensure and specialty board examinations for physicians nationwide and acts as a consultant for the CMA Certification Examination is:
   a. NBME
   b. CAAHEP
   c. ABHES
   d. AMTIE

3. How many test sites are there nationwide for the CMA examination?
   a. less than 250
   b. 250
   c. 250–500
   d. more than 500

4. In what months is the CMA examination offered?
   a. June and January
   b. September and January
   c. every month
   d. June, January, and October

5. A total of how many questions are on the CMA Certification Examination?
   a. 100
   b. 300
   c. 1,000
   d. It varies year to year.

6. How often does an RMA need to recertify?
   a. every year
   b. every 6 years
   c. every 5 years
   d. beginning in 2006, every 3 years

7. A total of how many points are required to recertify the CMA credential?
    a. 45
    b. 60
    c. 100
    d. 120

8. Which of the following are grounds for denial of eligibility for the CMA credential?
    a. unauthorized possession of the examination materials
    b. copying or permitting another to copy answers
    c. falsifying information required for admission to the examination
    d. all of the above

CASE STUDY

Michele Lucas is performing an externship at Inner City Health Care under the direction of office manager Jane O'Hara. Michele has purchased a certification review study guide and has taken the sample 120-question Certification Examination available from the AAMA. From her studies, she has determined that she needs more work in the area of collections and insurance processing. Part-time administrative medical assistant Karen Ritter is responsible for these duties at Inner City Health Care, under Jane's supervision.

Discuss the following:
1. How can Michele use her externship experience to help her concentrate on improving her skills in the area of collections and insurance processing?
2. What are your own personal strengths and weaknesses in preparing for the CMA Certification Examination? What can you do to improve your areas of weakness?

SELF-ASSESSMENT

1. Think of two different places where you could get continuing education credits.
    a. Investigate each one.
    b. Write up a paragraph of the benefits and disadvantages of each method for you in your lifestyle.

2. Find out when and where your local chapter meetings are held.
    a. Attend a meeting with a classmate.
    b. Discuss what you learned from the meeting.

3. What can you do to prepare for the National Certification Examination?
    a. Write a plan in which you determine how much time you have to prepare and what you will accomplish each week/month in preparation.
    b. Make a calendar showing the steps toward your examination date.
    c. Try to stick with the plan as you progress closer to the examination date.

POST-TEST

This is similar to the Pre-Test. Perform this test without looking at the book. This is just to see how well you have understood and can recall the information presented in this chapter after you have studied it and completed the workbook exercises. You will not be graded on this portion (other than the grade you give yourself), but this is an excellent preparation for your instructor's test. You may use this Post-Test to determine what areas you need to study more. Justify any "false" answers.

1. An RMA and a CMA have different bylaws and creeds. (T or F)

2. A CMA is a national credential, so he or she may work in any state. (T or F)

3. Three major areas included in the CMA examination are clinical, administrative, and transdisciplinary (general medical knowledge). (T or F)

4. Physicians recognize that their offices operate much more efficiently and effectively with professionally trained and formally educated personnel such as medical assistants. (T or F)

5. A CMA has to be a member of AAMA or currently employed to recertify. (T or F)

6. On meeting recertification requirements, the applicant will receive a dated seal to apply to their original certificate. (T or F)

7. Once a student has become a member of AAMA, he or she may stay at the student rate for two years after graduation. (T or F)

CERTIFICATION CRITERIA CHECKLIST

As you go through your education and training, keep in mind the national certification examination that you will take when you graduate. Each chapter of the textbook and workbook covers a different section of the examination criteria. To keep track of your preparation for the certification examination, turn to the back of this workbook and highlight the following CMA, RMA, or CMAS certification examination criteria (if you have already highlighted them from a previous chapter, put a check mark by the criteria):

CMA
D. Professionalism
    1. Displaying professional attitude
E. Communication
    4. Professional communication and behavior

RMA
I. General Medical Assisting Knowledge
    C. Medical Law
II. Administrative Medical Assisting
    C. Medical Receptionist/Secretarial/Clerical
        4. Oral and written communication

CMAS
1. Medical Assisting Foundation
    • Legal and ethical considerations
3. Medical Office Clerical Assisting
    • Communication

EVALUATION OF CHAPTER KNOWLEDGE

Skills	Student Self-Evaluation		
	Good	Average	Poor
I can describe approved methods of training.	___	___	___
I can differentiate between being certified and being registered.	___	___	___
I can identify the benefits of certification.	___	___	___
I understand the qualifications to sit for the AAMA Certification Examination.	___	___	___
I know when the AAMA Certification Examination is offered and the registration deadlines.	___	___	___
I can describe methods for obtaining Continuing Education Units.	___	___	___
I understand the recertification process and its importance.	___	___	___
I understand the importance of enhancing skills through continuing education and the importance of maintaining professional growth throughout my career as a medical assistant.	___	___	___

CHAPTER 25

Employment Strategies

CHAPTER PRE-TEST

Perform this test without looking at the book. This is just to see how well you have understood and can recall the information in this chapter after you have read it, but before you have completed the workbook exercises. You will not be graded on this portion (other than the grade you give yourself). Justify any "false" answers.

1. Positive thinking is one of the primary keys to success in planning your career and during your job search. (T or F)

2. Job leads from friends, relatives, and neighbors are not the most successful for potential employment opportunities. (T or F)

3. Poor appearance is a reason for employers not to hire a job seeker. (T or F)

4. Employers like it when you know it all. They appreciate it when you do not ask questions. (T or F)

5. You should never expect to receive a job from an office where you are an extern. (T or F)

6. When filling out an application, it is acceptable to leave answers blank or write "see résumé." (T or F)

7. You should always plan ahead and have all your information with you when picking up an application, just in case you are asked to fill it out right there. (T or F)

INTRODUCTION

Once medical assisting students have completed their studies, it is time for them to start a career in their chosen field. There are various employment strategies that will greatly aid in obtaining a quality position in an ambulatory care setting. It is important that the job applicant adopt a strategy for job finding that includes self-assessment, job analysis and research, and budgetary needs analysis. In addition, there are several techniques that can make a difference in the success of a job-finding mission. Résumé preparation is one of the essential ingredients of the job hunt. A well-constructed résumé summarizing your work, education, and volunteer experience will make a vital connection in the interviewer's mind between what you can do and how these skills can benefit the organization. The construction of the cover letter or completion of the application form is also an important step in the success of the job-search process. The cover letter introduces the applicant to the potential employer with the goal of obtaining an interview. Once you have obtained an interview, you can prepare for it by learning what to expect in an interview and how to increase your chances for success.

PERFORMANCE OBJECTIVES

After successful completion of this chapter you will be able to explain the medical terms related to employment strategies. You will be able to list the steps involved in analyzing and researching a job. You will be able to describe a contact tracker and its usefulness; give examples of accomplishment statements; differentiate among chronologic, functional, and targeted résumés, and decide when each is the most appropriate; and be able to describe the purpose and content of a cover letter. You will be able to demonstrate effective ways to anticipate and respond to interviewer's questions, and you will be able to describe appropriate appearance for an interview and appropriate behavior at the interview. You will be able to write a good résumé, cover letter, and follow-up letter and cite the benefits of taking the time to do all well. *The following statements are related to your learning objectives. Fill in the blanks in the following paragraph with the appropriate term(s)*

One important quality an (1) _____ looks for in an employee is his or her (2) _____. Beyond having a (3) _____ attitude, being successful in your search for a job (4) _____ positive thinking on your part. Having success at finding that perfect job requires (5) _____ many hours to job strategy tactics. To begin, you need to (6) _____ what you want in a job. Take the time to complete a (7) _____ worksheet, such as the one in the textbook, to help you focus on your needs. Identify your direct (8) _____ and your (9) _____ skills. Job leads can come from many areas, including your (10) _____ site. As part of the job search, contact many individuals and keep track of the details in a (11) _____. Résumés should be (12) _____ and concise. Yours should be short and (13) _____ to read and understand. Use statements that are (14) _____ and reflect confidence and portray you as a (15) _____. Use (16) _____ statements if you have them from your (17) _____ or work experience. References are important, and always ask (18) _____ before using someone's name as a (19) _____. Proofread, proofread, and (20) _____ your résumé. There are various résumé styles, such as (21) _____, (22) _____, and (23) _____. Decide which type is best suited for your needs. Applications should be neat, complete, and accurate. Never write (24) _____ on an application, even though that might be easier. If your (25) _____ and (26) _____ have created a favorable impression, you may be granted an (27) _____. Be sure to follow the simple rules of etiquette and display a (28) _____ manner and image at the interview. Writing a (29) _____ letter after the interview is an excellent way to be remembered.

VOCABULARY BUILDER

Find the words listed below that are misspelled; circle them, and then correctly spell them in the spaces provided. Then match each correct vocabulary term to the aspect of the job-seeking process that best describes it.

_____ 1. accomplishment statements

_____ 2. application form

_____ 3. application/cover letter

_____ 4. bullat point

_____ 5. carreer objective

_____ 6. cronological résumé

_____ 7. contact tracker

_____ 8. functional résumé

_____ 9. interview

_____ 10. power verbs

_____ 11. refrences

_____ 12. résumé

_____ 13. targeted résumé

_____

_____   _____   _____

A. Expresses your career goal and the position for which you are applying

B. Résumé format used to highlight specialty areas of accomplishments and strengths

C. A form devised by a prospective employer to collect information relative to qualifications, education, and experience in employment

D. Individuals who have known or worked with you long enough to make an honest assessment and recommendation regarding your background history

E. Résumé format used when focusing on a clear, specific job

F. A statement that begins with a power verb and gives a brief description of what you did and the demonstrable results that were produced

G. Asterisk or dot followed by a descriptive phrase

H. A written summary data sheet or brief account of your qualifications and progress in your chosen career

I. Action words used to describe your attributes and strengths

J. A letter used to introduce yourself and your résumé to a prospective employer with the goal of obtaining an interview

K. Résumé format used when you have employment experience

L. A meeting in which you discuss employment opportunities and strengths that you can bring to the organization

M. Form used to keep track of employment contact information, such as name of employer, name of contact person, address and telephone number, date of first contact, résumé sent, interview date, and follow-up information and dates

LEARNING REVIEW

1. A variety of references should be included on your résumé or listed on a separate sheet of paper that closely matches your résumé. Give the appropriate response to the following questions.

   A. Choose references who are well-respected and are _____.

   B. List three types of professional references that would make excellent reference choices.
      (1) _____ (2) _____ (3) _____

   C. Identify someone you know or have contact with who fits each professional reference type listed above.
      (1) _____ (2) _____ (3) _____

2. There are various styles of résumés that can be used, depending on your employment strengths and abilities. Each particular style has advantages and disadvantages, and can be used singly or in combination. In some cases, a medical facility may prefer a certain résumé style.

   A. Identify situations when using a targeted résumé is advantageous by circling the number next to the statements that apply.
      (1) You are just starting your career and have little experience, but you know what you want and you are clear about your capabilities.
      (2) You want to use one résumé for several different applications.
      (3) You are not clear about your abilities and accomplishments.
      (4) You can go in several directions, and you want a different résumé for each.
      (5) You are able to keep your résumé on a computer disk.

   B. Identify the situations in which using a chronologic résumé is advantageous by circling the number next to the statements that apply.
      (1) You have been in the same job for many years.
      (2) Your job history shows real growth and development.
      (3) You are trained and employed in highly traditional fields (health care, government).
      (4) You are looking for your first job.
      (5) You are staying in the same field as prior jobs.

   C. Identify the situations in which using a functional résumé is advantageous by circling the number next to the statements that apply.
      (1) You have extensive specialized experience.
      (2) Your most recent employers have been highly prestigious.
      (3) You have had a variety of different, apparently unconnected, work experiences.
      (4) You want to emphasize a management growth pattern.
      (5) Much of your work has been volunteer, freelance, or temporary.

3. If you are sending your résumé to a potential employer, you will need to mail a cover letter with it. A well-written cover letter introduces you, tells the reader why you are writing and what you are sending, highlights your qualifications and experience, and enhances the information on your résumé. There are numerous guidelines to follow when writing a cover letter for submission to a potential employer. List four guidelines that are essential when preparing an effective cover letter.

   (1) _____

   (2) _____

   (3) _____

   (4) _____

4. When Ellen Armstrong, CMA, began her job search she encountered several employers who required her to complete an application form. Ellen could recall six points that were particularly important when filling out a job application. List four items that are important when completing a job application.

   (1) _____

   (2) _____

   (3) _____

   (4) _____

5. A. Bob Thompson has an interview at Inner City Health Care for a new clinical medical assisting position. He is confident he has prepared well for the interview. On the way to the interview, Bob reminds himself of three principles he has learned about interviewing.

   (1) _____ before answering questions, trying to provide the information requested in a _____ manner.

   (2) _____ carefully so that you understand what information the interviewer is requesting.

   (3) _____ for _____ if you are uncertain.

   B. Bob Thompson also recalls that it is not appropriate to ask questions about certain subjects during a first interview, but instead to concentrate on the value and skills one can contribute to the organization. Name four items you should not ask questions about in a first interview.

   (1) _____   (3) _____

   (2) _____   (4) _____

CERTIFICATION REVIEW

These questions are designed to mimic the certification examinations. You can use these questions like a small "Certification Examination Study Guide," but this is not meant to take the place of the more extensive study guides. Use this portion to determine in what areas to concentrate your efforts when studying for the certification examination.

1. Telling your friends, family, personal physician, dentist, and ophthalmologist that you are looking for a position in health care is called:
   a. networking
   b. references
   c. professionalism
   d. critiquing

2. Summarizing employment is acceptable on a résumé if it is prior to how many years ago?
   a. 1 year
   b. 5 years
   c. 10 years
   d. 15 years

3. The type of résumé that should be developed by someone looking for their first job is a:
   a. targeted résumé
   b. chronologic résumé
   c. functional résumé
   d. objective résumé

4. Poise includes such things as:
   a. skill level
   b. confidence and appearance
   c. a and b
   d. none of the above

5. Providing a second opportunity to express your interest in an organization and a position may be done with a:
   a. cover letter
   b. recommendation letter
   c. follow-up letter
   d. strategic letter

CASE STUDY

You are the subject of this case study. Complete the Self-Evaluation Worksheet that follows. Use your answers to help you determine the working environment you are most interested in and that best suits you. The worksheet can become a useful tool when researching prospective employers to target for your exciting first job in the medical assisting profession.

SELF-EVALUATION WORKSHEET

Respond to the following questions honestly and sincerely. They are meant to assist you in self-assessment.

1. List your strongest attributes as related to people, data, or things.

   i.e., Interpersonal skills related to people

   Accuracy related to data

   Mechanical ability related to things

   _____ related to _____

   _____ related to _____

   _____ related to _____

2. List your three weakest attributes related to people, data, or things.

   _____ related to _____

   _____ related to _____

   _____ related to _____

3. How do you express yourself? excellent, good, fair, poor

   Orally _____ In writing _____

4. Do you work well as a leader of a group or team? Yes _____ No _____

5. Do you prefer to work alone and on your own? Yes _____ No _____

6. Can you work under stress/pressure? Yes _____ No _____

7. Do you enjoy new ideas and situations? Yes _____ No _____

8. Are you comfortable with routines/schedules? Yes _____ No _____

9. Which work setting do you prefer?

   Single-physician setting _____ Multiphysician setting _____

   Small clinic setting _____ Large clinic setting _____

   Single-specialty setting _____ Multispecialty setting _____

10. Are you willing to relocate? _____ Willing to travel? _____

SELF-ASSESSMENT

Pretend you are interviewing a recent graduate for a medical assisting position.

1. What questions would you want to know the answers to?

2. Would you want to know the answers to some illegal or unethical questions? Do you think there is a way to obtain that information without actually asking the questions?

3. Do you think you could determine the best person for the job by meeting him or her just once? What else might you do to get to know the person better or get to know his or her work style better?

POST-TEST

This is similar to the Pre-Test. Perform this test without looking at the book. This is just to see how well you have understood and can recall the information presented in this chapter after you have studied it and completed the workbook exercises. You will not be graded on this portion (other than the grade you give yourself), but this is an excellent preparation for your instructor's test. You may use this Post-Test to determine what areas you need to study more. Justify any "false" answers.

1. Positive thinking is a good thing, but it is not all that important to success in planning your career and during your job search. (T or F)

2. Job leads from friends, relatives, and neighbors are some of the most successful for potential employment opportunities. (T or F)

3. Professional appearance is one reason for employers to want to hire a job seeker. (T or F)

4. Employers do not expect that you will know it all. They appreciate it when you ask questions. (T or F)

5. Students often receive job offers from the office where they extern. (T or F)

6. When filling out an application, it is never acceptable to leave answers blank or write "see résumé." (T or F)

7. Plan ahead and have all your information with you when you pick up an application, just in case you are asked to fill it out right there. (T or F)

CERTIFICATION CRITERIA CHECKLIST

As you go through your education and training, keep in mind the national certification examination that you will take when you graduate. Each chapter of the textbook and workbook covers a different section of the examination criteria. To keep track of your preparation for the certification examination, turn to the back of this workbook and highlight the following CMA, RMA, or CMAS certification examination criteria (if you have already highlighted them from a previous chapter, put a check mark by the criteria):

CMA
D. Professionalism
    1. Displaying professional attitude
    2. Job readiness and seeking employment
E. Communication
    6. Interviewing techniques

RMA
I. General Medical Assisting Knowledge
    C. Medical Law
    E. Human Relations
II. Administrative Medical Assisting
    C. Medical Receptionist/Secretarial/Clerical
        4. Oral and written communication

CMAS
1. Medical Assisting Foundation
    • Legal and ethical considerations
    • Professionalism
3. Medical Office Clerical Assisting
    • Communication

EVALUATION OF CHAPTER KNOWLEDGE

Skills	Student Self-Evaluation		
	Good	Average	Poor
I can name the steps of job analysis and research.	____	____	____
I can describe the function and use of a contact tracker.	____	____	____
I can differentiate among chronologic, functional, and targeted résumés.	____	____	____
I can implement power words to compose accomplishment statements for résumés.	____	____	____
I know the purpose and content of a cover letter.	____	____	____
I can demonstrate effective behavior during interview sessions.	____	____	____
I understand the importance of displaying professionalism.	____	____	____
I can identify benefits of follow-up letters.	____	____	____
I use self-assessment techniques to determine optimal employment goals.	____	____	____

Case Studies

INTRODUCTION

This appendix presents six case studies designed to give you experience using medical office practice management software. Using *Medical Office Simulation Software (MOSS)*, you will enroll the patients and their family members using the information provided for each patient. To complete each case study, you will also need to create appointments, post procedure charges, bill insurance companies and individual patients, and post payments received by the office.

INSTALLING MOSS ON YOUR COMPUTER

1. Take the CD from the back of the Workbook that accompanies *Thomson Delmar Learning's Comprehensive Medical Assisting, Third Edition*, and place it into your CD-ROM drive.

2. The Medical Office Simulation Software should begin setup automatically. Follow the on-screen prompts to install MOSS, Access Runtime, and SnapShot Viewer.

3. If MOSS does not begin setup automatically, follow these instructions:

   - Double-click on My Computer.
   - Double-click the Control Panel icon.
   - Double-click Add/Remove Programs.
   - Click the Install button, and follow the on-screen prompts.

USING MEDICAL OFFICE SIMULATION SOFTWARE

When you finish installing MOSS, it will be accessible through the Start menu. Select Start → All Programs → Medical Office Simulation Software → MOSS to open the software. At the logon screen, click OK to enter MOSS. Your user name and password are already loaded for you. You may change your password after you have logged in, by going to the File Maintenance area of the software.

Menu Screen

In MOSS, the user will be oriented to the general functions of most practice management software. MOSS features a Main Menu screen consisting of buttons that provide access to specific areas. Alternatively, there is an icon bar along the top left to quickly access the areas of the software, or the user may choose to navigate the software by using the pull-down menus below the software title bar.

There are eight basic components common to most practice management software. These include:

- Patient Registration
- Appointment Scheduling
- Procedure Posting
- Insurance Billing
- Posting Payments
- Patient Billing

- Report Generation
- File Maintenance

Patient Registration

The patient registration area allows the user to input information about each patient in the practice, including demographic, Health Insurance Portability and Accountability Act (HIPAA), and medical insurance information. From the Main Menu screen, click on the Patient Registration button to search for a patient, or to add a new patient, using the command buttons along the bottom of the patient selection dialog box.

Appointment Scheduling

The appointment scheduling system enables the user to make appointments and also cancel, reschedule, and search for appointments. MOSS allows for block scheduling, as well as several print features including appointment cards and daily schedules.

Procedure Posting

In the procedure posting system, patient fees for services are applied, in addition to relevant information such as service dates and place of service information. When procedures are input into the procedure posting system, the software assigns the fee to be charged according to the fee schedule for the patient's insurance.

Insurance Billing

The insurance billing system is designed to prepare claims to be sent to insurance companies for the medical office to receive payment for services provided. MOSS allows the user to generate and print a paper claim or simulate sending the claim electronically.

Posting Payments and Patient Billing

In the posting payments system, the user may input payments received by the practice from patients or insurance companies, as well as enter adjustments to the account. Once the payment from the primary insurance company has been posted, the software can generate a claim to a secondary insurance company, if applicable, or generate a bill to be sent directly to the patient to collect the outstanding balance.

File Maintenance and User Help

The File Maintenance System is a utility area of the program that contains common information used by various systems within the software. It is also an area where the setup of the software system can be adjusted or customized.

Under the Help tab, the user can turn Feedback Mode and Balloon Help Mode on or off. Feedback mode will alert the user when essential fields have not been completed before allowing data to be saved. Balloon Help offers explanations, clarification, or reminders for certain fields.

System Requirements

- Pentium II, 500 MHz minimum; Pentium III, 1 GHz recommended
- Microsoft Windows® 98, ME, 2000, XP
- 400 MB hard disk
- 64 MB RAM required, 256 MB RAM recommended
- 800 × 600 monitor display
- MS Access® 2000 recommended (MS Access Runtime supplied on MOSS CD)

Technical Support

Technical Support at Thomson Delmar Learning is available from 8:30 AM to 5:30 PM Eastern Standard Time.

- Phone: (800) 477-3692
- Fax: (518) 881-1247
- E-mail: delmarhelp@thomson.com

CASE STUDY 1: DAVID AND LOIS FITZPATRICK

The Fitzpatrick family recently moved to Douglasville from Albany, NY. Mr. Fitzpatrick has taken a promotion with his employer, the NY State Department of Corrections, which required him to relocate to the central facility.

1. **Patient Registration.** Enroll David and Lois Fitzpatrick with the Douglasville Medicine Associates practice using MOSS.

TABLE 1 PATIENT REGISTRATION INFORMATION FOR DAVID AND LOIS FITZPATRICK

Physician	Dr. Schwartz	Dr. Schwartz
Last Name	Fitzpatrick	Fitzpatrick
First Name	David	Lois
Middle Initial	J	J
SSN (Social Security number)	999-12-4567	999-21-3457
Gender	M	F
Marital Status	Married	Married
Date of Birth	01/25/49	10/17/50
Address	625 Renaud Ave.	625 Renaud Ave.
City	Douglasville	Douglasville
State	NY	NY
ZIP	01234	01234
Home Phone	(123) 456-1318	(123) 456-1318
Employer/School	NY Department of Corrections	Randall Craig Associates, LLC
Address	452 Chain Link Fence Way	29 Commerce Way
City	Douglasville	Douglasville
State	NY	NY
ZIP	01234	01234
Work Phone	(123) 456-2100, Ext 472	(123) 676-1280, Ext 21
Referring Physician	Samantha Green, MD	Samantha Green, MD
Guarantor	Self	Spouse
Relationship to Patient	Self	Spouse
Insurance—Primary	Consumer One—HRA	Consumer One—HRA
Patient Relationship to Insured	Self	Spouse
Policy Holder Information		
Last Name	Self	Fitzpatrick
First Name		David
Date of Birth		10-25-1949
ID #	999-12-4567A	999-12-4567A
Policy Number	ABC37156564	ABC37156564
Group Number	NYDOC1000	NYDOC1000
Employer Name	NY Department of Corrections	NY Department of Corrections
PCP (primary care physician)	N/A	N/A
Insurance—Secondary	N/A	N/A
Additional Information	Your practice accepts assignment, the patient's signatures are on file, and this is an in-network/PAR.	Your practice accepts assignment, the patient's signatures are on file, and this is an in-network/PAR.

2. **Insurance Verification.** Whether new or established, it is essential to verify every patient's medical insurance. Using the Online Eligibility feature in MOSS, verify the insurance eligibility for David and Lois Fitzpatrick. View and print the report.

3. **Creating Appointments.**

   a. Today is November 4, 2004. Mr. Fitzpatrick is not accustomed to the water in this area of the country and suffers from intestinal distress. He called this morning to see the doctor as soon as possible. Schedule an appointment for him for this afternoon at 2:00 PM. He is a new patient and will need a comprehensive office visit for one hour. Be sure to check Mr. Fitzpatrick in on your appointment scheduler when he arrives for his office visit.

   b. Mrs. Fitzpatrick calls one week later and requests to see her doctor. She is not sure what is wrong with her; she just feels unusually tired. Mrs. Fitzpatrick is also a new patient and will need a comprehensive office visit for one hour. Schedule an appointment for Mrs. Fitzpatrick on November 11, 2004, at 9 AM. Be sure to check Mrs. Fitzpatrick in on your appointment scheduler when she arrives for her office visit.

4. **Posting Procedures.**

   a. Mr. Fitzpatrick was diagnosed with gastroenteritis and given a prescription. Post the charges for his comprehensive, 60-minute office visit (the reference number on his superbill is 5001). Dr. Schwartz has indicated on the superbill that Mr. Fitzpatrick

   is to return for a follow-up appointment in one week. Make a follow-up appointment for Mr. Fitzpatrick on November 12, 2004, at 11 AM.

   b. Mrs. Fitzpatrick's visit required her physician to perform a comprehensive history and examination. The physician ordered a blood sugar test, a routine urinalysis (UA) with Micro, a complete blood cell count (CBC) with differential, and a hematocrit. She was diagnosed with generalized weakness. Post the charges for her comprehensive, 60-minute office visit (the superbill reference number is 5043). Dr. Schwartz wants to see her again in two weeks for a follow-up appointment. Make a follow-up appointment for Mrs. Fitzpatrick on November 24, 2004, at 10:30 AM.

5. **Billing.**

   a. Neither Mr. nor Mrs. Fitzpatrick made a payment at the time of their visit.

   b. Using the Insurance Billing feature in MOSS, generate and submit electronic claims to the insurance company for Mr. and Mrs. Fitzpatrick's November 4 and 11 visits.

6. **Posting Insurance Payments.** A few weeks have gone by and you receive an explanation of benefits (EOB) with a check for both of the Fitzpatricks' claims. The insurance company has paid 100% of the billed items. Post the insurance payment on December 15, 2004, to the Fitzpatricks' accounts. The reference number for the Fitzpatricks' EOB is 99123350.

CASE STUDY 2: DIANE, ROBERT, AND HANNALEY MELLO

The Mello family was referred to your practice by Dr. Reed. The Mellos have recently switched insurance plans to receive more comprehensive medical coverage. Mr. Mello is a construction worker and his wife, Diane, is a waitress at a local family restaurant. They have a daughter, Hannaley, who is asthmatic and requires a broad spectrum of health care needs.

1. **Patient Registration.** Enroll the Mellos with the Douglasville Medicine Associates practice using MOSS.

TABLE 2 PATIENT REGISTRATION INFORMATION FOR THE MELLO FAMILY

Physician	Heath	Heath	Heath
Last Name	Mello	Mello	Mello
First Name	Robert	Diane	Hannaley
Middle Initial	J	E	
SSN	999-27-4321	999-27-8002	999-32-9730
Gender	M	F	F
Marital Status	Married	Married	Single
Date of Birth	09/23/70	04/18/71	06/17/95
Address	28 Barbara Lane	28 Barbara Lane	28 Barbara Lane
Apartment/Unit			
City	Douglasville	Douglasville	Douglasville
State	NY	NY	NY
ZIP	01234	01234	01234
Home Phone	(123) 676-0332	(123) 676-0332	(123) 676-0332
Employer/School	Triple A Contractors	Grandma's Family Restaurant	Morton Elementary School
Address	435 Rhode Island Ave.	273 President Ave.	231 Main Road
City	Douglasville	Douglasville	Douglasville
State	NY	NY	NY
ZIP	01234	01234	01234
Work Phone	(123) 676-4353	(123) 676-0223	(123) 677-3210
Referring Physician	Reed	Reed	Reed
Guarantor	Self	Robert Mello	Robert Mello
Relationship to Patient	Self	Spouse	Child
Insurance—Primary	Signal HMO	Signal HMO	Signal HMO
Patient Relationship to Insured	Self	Spouse	Child
Policy Holder Information			
Last Name	Self	Mello	Mello
First Name		Robert	Robert
Date of Birth		09/23/70	09/23/70
ID #	999-27-4321BB	999-27-4321BB	999-27-4321BB
Policy Number	DE48329J	DE48329J	DE48329J
Group Number	N/A	N/A	N/A
Employer Name	Triple A Contractors	Triple A Contractors	Triple A Contractors
PCP	N/A	N/A	N/A
Copayment	$10.00	$10.00	$10.00
Insurance—Secondary	N/A	N/A	N/A
Additional Information	Your practice accepts assignment, the patient's signatures are on file, and this is an in-network/PAR.	Your practice accepts assignment, the patient's signatures are on file, and this is an in-network/PAR.	Your practice accepts assignment, the patient's signatures are on file, and this is an in-network/PAR.

2. **Insurance Verifications.** Whether new or established, it is essential to verify every patient's medical insurance. Using the Online Eligibility feature, verify the insurance eligibility for the Mellos. View and print the report.

3. **Creating Appointments.** Today is November 4, 2005. Mr. Mello called to make a same-day appointment. He has experienced persistent loose stools and vomiting. He has a temperature of 101.2°F. His wife and daughter are experiencing similar symptoms. Create appointments for all three patients at 3:00 PM, 3:15 PM, and 3:30 PM. Be sure to check all three patients in on your appointment scheduler when they arrive for their office visits.

4. **Posting Procedures.** All of the Mellos received a problem-focused history and examination.

(*Hint:* Remember that the Mellos are new patients.) All were diagnosed with gastritis. Post the charges to each member's account. The superbill reference numbers are 5011, 5012, and 5013. Because Mrs. Mello exhibited the most severe symptoms, the doctor asked that she return in two weeks for a follow-up examination. Make a follow-up appointment for Mrs. Mello on November 16, 2004, at 2 PM.

5. **Billing and Payments.**

   a. Collect the copayment of $10.00 for each patient. Mr. Mello writes check number 1088 for $30.00.

   b. Prepare insurance claim forms and send electronically to their insurance company.

CASE STUDY 3: SEAN AND MANUELLA GILBERTSON

There are occasions when your providers will see patients in outside facilities such as in the hospital or a skilled nursing facility. When this occurs for new patients, it is essential that as much information as possible is gathered by the provider and verified and supplemented by the medical office staff. In the fol-

lowing case study, Dr. Heath made his weekly visit to the Retirement Inn Nursing Home where he met with all his patients. Today, he also saw the Gilbertsons, who recently were entered into care at that facility.

1. **Patient Registration.** Enroll the Gilbertsons with the Douglasville Medicine Associates practice using MOSS.

TABLE 3 PATIENT REGISTRATION INFORMATION FOR SEAN AND MANUELLA GILBERTSON

Physician	Heath	Heath
Last Name	Gilbertson	Gilbertson
First Name	Sean	Manuella
Middle Initial	G	A
SSN	999-11-1114	999-99-0003
Gender	M	F
Marital Status	Married	Married
Date of Birth	03/11/39	10/17/39
Address	438 Courtship Ave.	438 Courtship Ave.
Apartment/Unit		
City	Douglasville	Douglasville
State	NY	NY
ZIP	01234	01234
Home Phone	(123) 678-6765	(123) 678-6765
Employer/School	Retired	Retired
Referring Physician	Reed	Reed
Guarantor	Self	Spouse
Relationship to Patient	Self	Spouse
Insurance—Primary	Medicare—Statewide Corp	Medicare—Statewide Corp
Patient Relationship to Insured	Self	Spouse
Policy Holder Information	Self	Spouse
Last Name		Gilbertson
First Name		Sean
Date of Birth		03/11/1939
ID #	999-11-1114	999-11-1114
Policy Number		
Group Number		
Employer Name		
PCP		
Insurance—Secondary	Medicaid	Medicaid
Patient Relationship to Insured	Self	Self
Policy Holder Information	Self	Self
Last Name		
First Name		
Date of Birth		
ID #	999-11-1114M	999-99-0003M
Policy Number		
Group Number		
Employer Name		
PCP Name (if applicable)		
Additional Information	Your practice accepts assignment, the patient's signatures are on file, and Dr. Heath is a Medicare and Medicaid participating provider.	Your practice accepts assignment, the patient's signatures are on file, and Dr. Heath is a Medicare and Medicaid participating provider.

2. **Insurance Verifications.** Whether new or established, it is essential to verify every patient's medical insurance. Using the Online Eligibility feature, verify the insurance eligibility for the Gilbertsons. View and print the report.

3. **Appointments.** Today is November 2, 2005. The Gilbertsons are residents of the Retirement Inn Nursing Home. Dr. Heath makes weekly visits to his patients in the nursing home on Tuesday mornings. Today, he saw the Gilbertsons starting at 10:30 in the morning. They recently were admitted and are now under Dr. Heath's care.

4. **Posting Procedures.** Dr. Heath provided a Level 5 new patient comprehensive examination for each patient. For Mr. Gilbertson, the examination focused on his cardiac pulmonary disease; for Mrs. Gilbertson, it focused on her insulin-dependent diabetes. (*Hint:* Dr. Heath reported the procedures on an Outside Service log, as numbers 003 and 004.)

5. **Billing.**

   a. There is no copayment due at the time of service.

   b. Using the Insurance Billing feature, generate and print a paper claim to submit to Medicare.

6. **Posting Insurance Payments.** Five weeks have gone by and you receive an EOB for both Mr. and Mrs. Gilbertson, with a check for $404.80 ($202.40 for each account) and a statement that the balance for the unpaid portion has been submitted to Medicaid. Post the insurance payment on December 8, 2004, to the Gilbertson's accounts, using 972211101 as the reference number.

7. **Billing Secondary Insurance.** Using the Insurance Billing feature, generate and transmit an electronic claim to Medicaid, the Gilbertsons' secondary insurance.

CASE STUDY 4: STEPHANIE M. ROBERTSON

Stephanie Robertson is an emancipated minor who seeks free or reduced-fee care at your clinic. She has no insurance and little money in the bank. She has applied for state aid, but has not yet received it.

1. **Patient Registration.** Enroll Stephanie Robertson with the Douglasville Medicine Associates practice using MOSS.

TABLE 4   PATIENT REGISTRATION INFORMATION FOR STEPHANIE ROBERTSON

Physician	Schwartz
Last Name	Robertson
First Name	Stephanie
Middle Initial	M
SSN	999-98-2020
Gender	F
Marital Status	Single
Date of Birth	12/11/87
Address	1318 Renaud St.
Apartment/Unit	12A
City	Douglasville
State	NY
ZIP	01234
Home Phone	(123) 677-2525
Employer/School	Sloppy Joe's Burgers
Address	38 Main Road
City	Douglasville
State	NY
ZIP	01234
Work Phone	(123) 456-2708
Referring Physician	None
Guarantor	Self-Pay
Relationship to Patient	Self
Insurance—Primary	Self-Pay
Additional Information	Self-Pay

2. **Creating Appointments.** Today is November 5, 2005. Stephanie Robertson makes a 45-minute appointment for November 12, 2004, at 10:30 AM. She says that the reason is "personal." Be sure to check Ms. Robertson in on your appointment scheduler when she arrives for her office visit.

3. **Posting Procedures.** Dr. Schwartz performs a Level 4 new patient examination. He also performs a routine pelvic examination, draws blood for a Venereal Disease Research Laboratory (VDRL) test, a mononucleosis screen, and a UA with microscopy. She was seen for abdominal pain. Post the charges to her account, using 6112 as the superbill reference number.

4. **Billing.**

   a. There is no copayment due.

   b. You collect $20.00 in cash from the patient today and make arrangements to bill her $50.00 per month until the bill is paid. Post this payment to Ms. Robertson's account.

5. **Patient Billing.** Prepare Ms. Robertson's first billing statement on December 8, 2004. Be sure to include a message on her patient statement, per your agreement, to remit December's payment of $50.00.

6. **Posting Payments.** On December 17, 2004, you receive check number 151 from Ms. Robertson for the amount of $50.00. Post this amount to her account.

CASE STUDY 5: MARY AND HENRY SMITH

Occasionally there will be accounts where the guarantor and the insured party are not one and the same. This is the case with Mr. and Mrs. Smith. Mr. Smith is the unemployed spouse of Mrs. Smith, who is a real estate broker of a very successful firm. Although Mrs. Smith is the insured party, her husband is the guarantor of the account.

1. **Patient Registration.** Enroll the Smiths with the Douglasville Medicine Associates practice using MOSS. Be sure to identify Mr. Smith as the account guarantor.

TABLE 5 PATIENT REGISTRATION INFORMATION FOR HENRY AND MARY SMITH

Physician	Heath	Heath
Last Name	Smith	Smith
First Name	Henry	Mary
Middle Initial	E	M
SSN	999-00-1110	999-10-3333
Gender	M	F
Marital Status	Married	Married
Date of Birth	02/14/69	09/18/70
Address	82 Hartwell St.	82 Hartwell St.
Apartment/Unit		
City	Douglasville	Douglasville
State	NY	NY
ZIP	01234	01234
Home Phone	(123) 678-2740	(123) 678-2740
Employer/School	Unemployed	Homestead Realty, LLC
Address		4832 Home Owner Way
City		Douglasville
State		NY
ZIP		01234
Work Phone		(123) 467-4983, Ext 21
Referring Physician	Green	Green
Guarantor	Self	Spouse
Relationship to Patient	Self	Spouse
Insurance—Primary	Flexi-Health PPO	Flexi-Health PPO
Patient Relationship to Insured	Spouse	Self
Policy Holder Information		
Last Name	Smith	Self
First Name	Mary	
Date of Birth	09/18/70	
ID #	999-10-3333	999-10-3333
Policy Number		
Group Number		
Employer	Homestead Realty, LLC	Homestead Realty, LLC
PCP		
Copayment	$20.00	$20.00
Insurance—Secondary	N/A	N/A
Additional Information	Your practice accepts assignment, the patient's signatures are on file, and Dr. Heath is a participating provider of her insurance plan.	Your practice accepts assignment, the patient's signatures are on file, and Dr. Heath is a participating provider of her insurance plan.

2. **Insurance Verifications.** Whether new or established, it is essential to verify every patient's medical insurance. Using the Online Eligibility feature, verify the insurance eligibility for the Smiths. View and print the report.

3. **Creating Appointments.**

   a. Today is November 15, 2004. The Smiths have registered with your practice and want to make appointments for a general checkup. However, Mr. Smith suspects he has an upper respiratory infection of some sort, and Mrs. Smith just simply feels over-tired and run down.

   b. They request an appointment during their lunch time at about 12:30 PM. You realize that this conflicts with your appointment matrix. Try to accommodate their needs. If unable to do so, schedule them in a time slot just before or after Dr. Heath's lunch.

4. **Posting Procedures.**

   a. Dr. Heath provided a Level 5 new patient comprehensive examination for each patient.

   b. Mr. Smith was diagnosed with acute bronchitis, and Mrs. Smith was diagnosed with generalized weakness, most likely due to stress. Post the charges to their accounts using 6225 and 6226 as the reference numbers.

5. **Billing and Payments.**

   a. There is $20.00 copayment for each patient. However, Mr. Smith will be paying cash for all of his charges. Post the cash payment for Mr. Smith.

   b. Post Mrs. Smith's $20.00 copayment to her account, and use the Insurance Billing feature to bill the remainder to her insurance. Generate and submit an electronic claim to Mrs. Smith's insurance company.

6. **Posting Payments.** Five weeks have gone by and you receive and EOB with a check from Flexi-Health for the balance of Mrs. Smith's account. Post the insurance check on December 20, 2004, to Mrs. Smith's account.

CASE STUDY 6: VITO AND ERMALINDA WILLIAMS

It is always nice when things work the way in which they are designed. All too often, though, they do not. Patients will cancel appointments, change appointments, or ask if they can bring a dependent beneficiary to the appointment to be seen as well. Occasionally medical office staff may fail to enter an appointment or even make an appointment for the wrong date, time, or provider. When these occurrences happen, they must be reflected and/or corrected in the medical office practice management software.

Vito and Ermalinda Williams are an older adult couple who depend on family members for help. Of particular help is their daughter, who has been their most reliable source of support. In fact, they generally make their appointments based on their daughter's availability.

1. **Patient Registration.** Enroll the Mr. and Mrs. Williams with the Douglasville Medicine Associates practice using MOSS. Note that Mr. Williams is the account guarantor. However, each patient has their individual Medicare and Medicaid medical coverage.

2. **Insurance Verifications.** Whether new or established, it is essential to verify every patient's medical insurance. Using the Online Eligibility feature, verify the insurance eligibility for Mr. and Mrs. Williams. View and print the report.

3. **Creating Appointments.**

   a. Today is November 15, 2004. Mr. Williams calls to make an appointment for both he

and his wife for tomorrow, if possible. Both have similar symptoms of slight nausea, stomach pains, and chills.

   b. Today is November 16, 2004. Mr. Williams calls to say his daughter will not be able to bring him and his wife to the office today. He also states the symptoms have not worsened, and that they would like to be seen tomorrow, November 17, 2004. NOTE: For the purposes of this scenario, assume their assigned physician, Dr. Schwartz, is not available. Make an appointment for Mr. and Mrs. Williams to see Dr. Heath.

4. **Posting Procedures.**

   a. Dr. Heath provided a Level 2 new patient examination for each patient.

   b. Mr. and Mrs. Williams were diagnosed with gastritis and mild dehydration.

5. **Billing.**

   a. There is no copayment for either patient; however, it is not known if either of them has met their annual deductible.

   b. Use the Insurance Billing feature to generate and print a paper claim for all charges to Medicare for both patients.

6. **Rebilling.** As of December 30, 2004, no checks have been received from Medicare. Rebill the insurance claims for both Vito and Ermalinda Williams.

TABLE 6   PATIENT REGISTRATION INFORMATION FOR VITO AND ERMALINDA WILLIAMS

Physician	Schwartz	Heath
Last Name	Williams	Williams
First Name	Vito	Ermalinda
Middle Initial	A	A
SSN	999-99-1110	999-99-3333
Sex	M	F
Marital Status	Married	Married
Date of Birth	10/17/41	12/25/40
Address	49 Renaud St.	49 Renaud St.
Apartment/Unit	Unit 27-A	Unit 27-A
City	Douglasville	Douglasville
State	NY	NY
ZIP	01234	01234
Home Phone	(123) 679-3636	(123) 679-3636
Employer/School	Retired	Retired
Address		
City		
State		
ZIP		
Work Phone		
Referring Physician	Brennen	Brennen
Guarantor	Self	Spouse
Relationship to Patient	Self	Spouse
Insurance—Primary	Medicare Statewide Corp	Medicare Statewide Corp
Patient Relationship to Insured	Self	Self
Policy Holder Information	Self	Self
Last Name		
First Name		
Date of Birth		
ID #	999-99-1110A	999-99-3333A
Policy Number		
Group Number		
Employer Name		
PCP		
Insurance—Secondary		
Plan Name	Medicaid	Medicaid
Patient Relationship to Insured	Self	Self
Policy Holder Information	Self	Self
Last Name		
First Name		
Date of Birth		
ID #	999-99-1110B	999-99-3333B
Policy Number		
Group Number		
Employer Name		
PCP		
Additional Information	Your practice accepts assignment, the patient's signatures are on file, and Dr. Heath is a participating provider of both Medicare and Medicaid plans.	Your practice accepts assignment, the patient's signatures are on file, and Dr. Heath is a participating provider of both Medicare and Medicaid plans.

Certification Criteria Checklists

Use these checklists to keep track of where in your studies you have learned the skills and criteria listed under the examination criteria. You may choose either the AAMA Certified Medical Assistant Certification/Recertification Examination Content Outline, the AMT Registered Medical Assistant Certification Examination Content, or the AMT Certified Medical Administrative Specialist Examination Competencies. You will find that many skills will be covered in multiple courses/chapters. This checklist will help you determine which areas you might need to cover in more detail as you prepare for your certification examination.

AAMA Certified Medical Assistant Certification/ Recertification Examination Content Outline	Workbook Checklist
I. A-F GENERAL	
A. MEDICAL TERMINOLOGY	
1. Word building and definitions	
2. Uses of terminology	
B. ANATOMY AND PHYSIOLOGY	
1. Body as a whole, including multiple systems	
2. Systems, including structure, function, related conditions and diseases	
C. PSYCHOLOGY	
1. Basic principles	
2. Developmental stages of the life cycle	
3. Hereditary, cultural and environmental influences on behavior	
4. Defense mechanisms	
D. PROFESSIONALISM	
1. Displaying professional attitude	
2. Job readiness and seeking employment	
3. Performing within ethical boundaries	
4. Maintaining confidentiality	
5. Working as a team member to achieve goals	

AAMA Certified Medical Assistant Certification/ Recertification Examination Content Outline	Workbook Checklist
E. COMMUNICATION	
1. Adapting communication to an individual's ability to understand (e.g., patients with special needs)	
2. Recognizing and responding to verbal and nonverbal communication	
3. Patient instruction	
4. Professional communication and behavior	
5. Evaluating and understanding communication	
6. Interviewing techniques	
7. Receiving, organizing, prioritizing and transmitting information	
8. Telephone techniques	
9. Fundamental writing skills	
F. MEDICOLEGAL GUIDELINES & REQUIREMENTS	
1. Licenses and accreditation	
2. Legislation	
3. Documentation/reporting	
4. Releasing medical information	
5. Physician-patient relationship	
II. G-Q ADMINISTRATIVE	
G. DATA ENTRY	
1. Keyboard fundamentals and functions	
2. Formats	
3. Proofreading	
H. EQUIPMENT	
1. Equipment operation	
2. Maintenance and repairs	
I. COMPUTER CONCEPTS	
1. Computer components	
2. Care and maintenance of computer	
3. Computer applications	
4. Internet services	
J. RECORDS MANAGEMENT	
1. Needs, purposes and terminology of filing systems	
2. Process for filing documents	
3. Organization of patient's medical record	
4. Filing guidelines	
5. Medical records	
K. SCREENING AND PROCESSING MAIL	
1. US Postal Service	
2. Private services	
3. Postal machine/meter	
4. Processing incoming mail	
5. Preparing outgoing mail	

AAMA Certified Medical Assistant Certification/ Recertification Examination Content Outline	Workbook Checklist
L. SCHEDULING AND MONITORING APPOINTMENTS	
1. Utilizing appointment schedules/types	
2. Appointment guidelines	
3. Appointment protocol	
M. RESOURCE INFORMATION AND COMMUNITY SERVICES	
1. Services available	
2. Appropriate referrals	
3. Follow-up	
4. Patient advocate	
N. MANAGING PHYSICIAN'S PROFESSIONAL SCHEDULE AND TRAVEL	
1. Arranging meetings (e.g., dates, facilities, accommodations)	
2. Scheduling travel	
3. Integrating meetings and travel with office schedule	
O. MANAGING THE OFFICE	
1. Maintaining the physical plant	
2. Equipment and supply inventory	
3. Maintaining liability coverage	
4. Time management	
P. OFFICE POLICIES AND PROCEDURES	
1. Patient information booklet	
2. Patient education	
3. Instructions for patients with special needs	
4. Personnel manual	
5. Policy and procedures manuals/protocols	
6. Compliance plan	
Q. MANAGING PRACTICE FINANCES	
1. Bookkeeping systems (e.g., single, double entry, pegboard, computer)	
2. Coding systems	
3. Third-party billing	
4. Accounting and banking procedures	
5. Employee payroll	
III. R-Z CLINICAL	
R. PRINCIPLES OF INFECTION CONTROL	
1. Principles of asepsis	
2. Aseptic technique	
3. Disposal of biohazardous material	
4. Practice Standard Precautions	
S. TREATMENT AREA	
1. Equipment preparation and operation	
2. Principles of operation	
3. Restocking supplies	
4. Preparing/maintaining treatment areas	
5. Safety precautions	

AAMA Certified Medical Assistant Certification/ Recertification Examination Content Outline	Workbook Checklist
T. PATIENT PREPARATION AND ASSISTING THE PHYSICIAN	
1. Performing telephone and in-person screening	
2. Vital signs	
3. Examinations	
4. Procedures	
5. Explanation and instructions	
6. Instruments, supplies and equipment	
U. PATIENT HISTORY INTERVIEW	
1. Components of patient history	
2. Documentation guidelines	
V. COLLECTING AND PROCESSING SPECIMENS; DIAGNOSTIC TESTING	
1. Methods of collection	
2. Processing specimens	
3. Quality control	
4. Performing selected tests	
5. Vision testing	
6. Hearing testing	
7. Respiratory testing	
8. Medical imaging	
W. PREPARING AND ADMINISTERING MEDICATIONS	
1. Pharmacology	
2. Preparing and administering oral and parenteral medications	
3. Prescriptions	
4. Maintain medication and immunization records	
5. Medical disposal	
6. Principles of IV therapy	
X. EMERGENCIES	
1. Preplanned action	
2. Assessment and triage	
Y. FIRST AID	
1. Establishing and maintaining an airway	
2. Identifying and responding to:	
3. Signs and symptoms	
4. Management	
Z. NUTRITION	
1. Basic principles	
2. Special needs	

AMT Registered Medical Assistant Certification Examination Content	Workbook Checklist
I. GENERAL MEDICAL ASSISTING KNOWLEDGE	
A. ANATOMY AND PHYSIOLOGY	
1. Body systems	
2. Disorders and diseases	
B. MEDICAL TERMINOLOGY	
1. Word parts	
2. Definitions	
3. Common abbreviations and symbols	
4. Spelling	
C. MEDICAL LAW	
1. Medical law	
2. Licensure, certification, and registration	
3. Terminology	
D. MEDICAL ETHICS	
1. Principles of medical ethics and ethical conduct	
E. HUMAN RELATIONS	
1. Patient relations	
2. Interpersonal relations	
F. PATIENT EDUCATION	
1. Patient instruction	
2. Patient resource materials	
3. Documentation	
4. Understand and utilize proper documentation of patient encounters/instruction	
II. ADMINISTRATIVE MEDICAL ASSISTING	
A. INSURANCE	
1. Terminology	
2. Plans	
3. Claims	
4. Coding	
5. Insurance finance applications	
B. FINANCE/BOOKKEEPING	
1. Terminology	
2. Patient billing	
3. Collections	
4. Fundamental medical office accounting procedures	
5. Banking procedures	
6. Employee payroll	
7. Financial mathematics	
C. MEDICAL RECEPTIONIST/SECRETARIAL/CLERICAL	
1. Terminology	
2. Reception	
3. Scheduling	
4. Oral and written communication	

AMT Registered Medical Assistant Certification Examination Content	Workbook Checklist
5. Records and chart management	
6. Transcription and dictation	
7. Supplies and equipment management	
8. Computer applications	
9. Office safety	
III. CLINICAL MEDICAL ASSISTING	
A. ASEPSIS	
1. Terminology	
2. Bloodborne pathogens and Universal Precautions	
3. Medical asepsis	
4. Surgical asepsis	
B. STERILIZATION	
1. Terminology	
2. Sanitation	
3. Disinfection	
4. Sterilization	
5. Recordkeeping	
C. INSTRUMENTS	
1. Identification	
2. Instrument use	
3. Care and handling	
D. VITAL SIGNS	
1. Terminology	
2. Blood pressure	
3. Pulse	
4. Respirations	
5. Temperature	
6. Mensurations	
E. PHYSICAL EXAMINATIONS	
1. Medical history	
2. Patient positions	
3. Methods of examination	
4. Specialty examinations: identify examination procedures in specialty practices	
5. Visual acuity	
6. Allergy	
7. Terminology	
F. CLINICAL PHARMACOLOGY	
1. Terminology	
2. Parenteral medications	
3. Prescriptions	
4. Drugs	
G. MINOR SURGERY	
1. Surgical supplies	
2. Surgical procedures	

AMT Registered Medical Assistant Certification Examination Content	Workbook Checklist
H. THERAPEUTIC MODALITIES	
1. Modalities	
2. Alternate therapies	
3. Patient instruction	
I. LABORATORY PROCEDURES	
1. Safety	
2. Clinical Laboratory Improvement Amendments (CLIA '88)	
3. Employ Quality Control program	
4. Laboratory equipment	
5. Laboratory testing	
6. Terminology	
J. ELECTROCARDIOGRAPHY (ECG)	
1. Standard 12-lead ECG	
2. Mounting techniques	
3. Identify other ECG procedures	
K. FIRST AID AND EMERGENCY RESPONSE	
1. First aid procedures	
2. Legal responsibilities	

AMT Certified Medical Administrative Specialist Examination Competencies	Workbook Checklist
1. MEDICAL ASSISTING FOUNDATION	
Medical terminology	
Anatomy and physiology	
Legal and ethical considerations	
Professionalism	
2. BASIC CLINICAL MEDICAL OFFICE ASSISTING	
Basic health history interview	
Basic charting	
Vital signs and measurements	
Asepsis in the medical office	
Examination preparation	
Medical office emergencies	
Basic pharmacology	
3. MEDICAL OFFICE CLERICAL ASSISTING	
Appointment management and scheduling	
Reception	
Communication	
Patient information and community resources	
4. MEDICAL RECORDS MANAGEMENT	
Systems	
Procedures	
Confidentiality	
5. HEALTH CARE INSURANCE PROCESSING, CODING AND BILLING	
Insurance processing	
Insurance coding	
Insurance billing and finances	
6. MEDICAL OFFICE FINANCIAL MANAGEMENT	
Fundamental financial management	
Patient accounts	
Banking	
Payroll	
7. MEDICAL OFFICE INFORMATION PROCESSING	
Fundamentals of computing	
Medical office computer applications	
8. MEDICAL OFFICE MANAGEMENT	
Office communications	
Business organizational management	
Human resources	
Safety	
Supplies and equipment	
Physical office plant	
Risk management and quality assurance	